Forty Days

I0885352

Forty Days: Quarantine and the Traveller, c. 1700–1900 provides a timely reminder that no traveller in past centuries could return from the East without spending up to 40 days in a lazaretto to ensure that no symptoms of plague were developing. Quarantine was performed in virtual prisons ranging from mud huts in the Danube basin to a converted fort on Malta, evoking every emotion from hatred and hostility through to resignation and even contentment. Drawing on the diaries and journals of some 300 men and women of many nationalities over more than two centuries, the author describes the inadequate accommodation, poor food and crushing boredom experienced by detainees. The book also draws attention to comradeship, sickness and death in detention, as well as Casanova's unique ability to do what he did best even in the lazaretto of Ancona. Other well-known detainees included Hans Christian Andersen, Mark Twain and Sir Walter Scott. Lavishly illustrated, the work includes a gazetteer of 49 lazarettos in Europe and Asia Minor, with inmates' comments on each. This book will appeal to all those interested in the history of medicine and the history of travel.

Dr John Booker, F.R.Hist.S., is an independent scholar based in Devon.

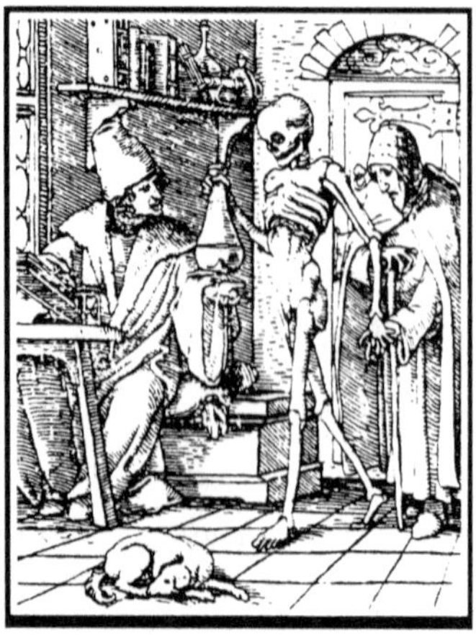

The History of Medicine in Context

Series Editors: Andrew Cunningham
(Department of History and Philosophy of Science, University of Cambridge)
Ole Peter Grell
(Department of History, Open University)

TITLES IN THE SERIES INCLUDE

The Afterlife of the Leiden Anatomical Collections
Hands On, Hands Off
Hieke Huistra

Civic Medicine
Physician, Polity, and Pen in Early Modern Europe
Edited by J. Andrew Mendelsohn, Annemarie Kinzelbach, and Ruth Schilling

Authority, Gender, and Midwifery in Early Modern Italy
Contested Deliveries
Jennifer F. Kosmin

Forty Days
Quarantine and the Traveller, c. 1700–1900
John Booker

For more information about this series, please visit: www.routledge.com/The-History-of-Medicine-in-Context/book-series/HMC

Forty Days

Quarantine and the Traveller, c. 1700–1900

John Booker

Routledge
Taylor & Francis Group
LONDON AND NEW YORK

First published 2022
by Routledge
2 Park Square, Milton Park, Abingdon, Oxon OX14 4RN

and by Routledge
605 Third Avenue, New York, NY 10158

Routledge is an imprint of the Taylor & Francis Group, an informa business

British Library Cataloguing-in-Publication Data
A catalogue record for this book is available from the British Library

Library of Congress Cataloging-in-Publication Data
A catalog record for this book has been requested

ISBN: 978-1-032-05034-8 (hbk)
ISBN: 978-1-032-05035-5 (pbk)
ISBN: 978-1-003-19573-3 (ebk)

DOI: 10.4324/9781003195733

Typeset in Sabon
by Apex CoVantage, LLC

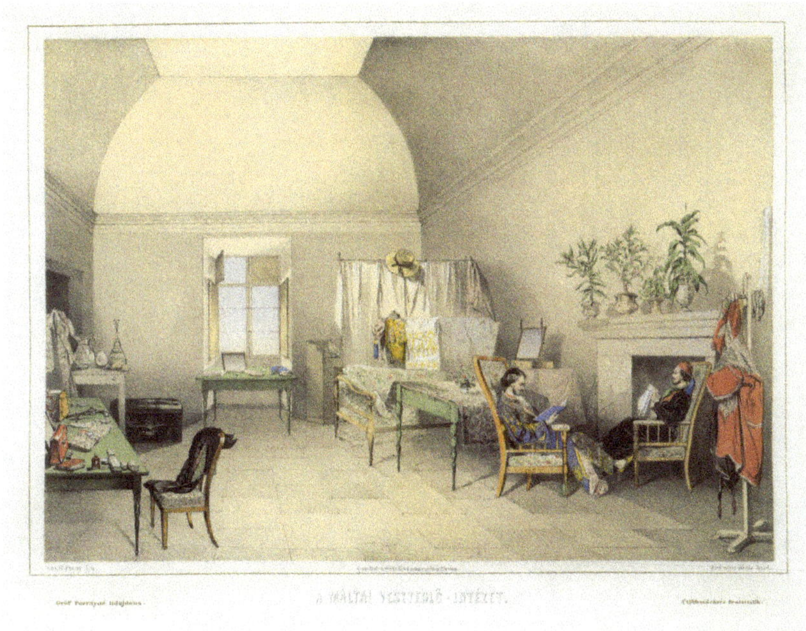

Frontispiece. Travellers whiling away the hours in the quarantine station at Malta. Any contemporary view within a lazaretto is remarkably rare.

Source: © The British Library Board, Tab. 1237.a. plate XIX

Contents

Illustrations

Maps

Acknowledgements

Research for this study was done when internet sources had not been developed to anything like the present level. I have spent countless hours in the London Library and the British Library, and to both institutions I tender my gratitude and affection. Staff at the Wellcome Library have been very helpful in guiding me to new shelves since the library's relocation. From the American School of Classical Studies at Athens, Aliki Asvesta sent me useful information on quarantine at Malta taken from an unpublished narrative in the Gennadius Library. Mrs Ann Mitchell received me hospitably in the Archives of Woburn Abbey, in connection with the travel records of the 6th Duke of Bedford, and Nicola Allen, archivist, has helpfully given me up-to-date references. The Trustees of the Bedford Estates have been kind enough to agree to the use of the material. The Manuscripts Department of Cambridge University Library gave me profitable access to the Kinglake papers. Among other repositories, I appreciated the facilities in Birmingham City Library, Somerset Record Office (now within the South West Heritage Trust) and University College London. In terms of the artwork, I have benefited yet again from the wisdom and experience of my friend Leo Maggs. My last words of gratitude must be reserved for my wife, Pam, who has been as tolerant as ever of her husband's abstruse interests.

The cover picture, frontispiece and illustrations 1, 38, 41, 42 and 44 are copyrighted and reproduced by kind permission of The British Library Board (see captions).

Author's note

Throughout this work the spelling of any place name corresponds with the usage during the period being discussed, which may represent its anglicized form. The modern spelling is usually given in the Gazetteer section. Likewise, the identity of the country in which that place is located, or by which it was controlled, is given in its historical context.

Glossary

Bill of health document given to a ship's master (very occasionally to individual travellers) by a consular official at the port of departure, explaining whether or not the locality was free of disease. The main types were 'clean', signifying all was well, or 'foul', indicating an active infection, but there were intermediate bills (having little relevance to the traveller) which identified the health of the hinterland with more precision.

Contagionism doctrine that disease, typically plague, was transmitted literally by touch. The vociferous opposing lobby was known as anti-contagionism.

Depuration the cleansing of a cargo by airing.

Lazaretto corruption of Italian word *lazzaretto* (fever hospital), signifying a building used for the quarantine of passengers and the airing of goods.

Parlatorio room attached to a lazaretto where inmates could converse at a distance with visitors or buy market wares.

Pratique the release of a ship or person from all restrictions on account of quarantine; often called **free pratique**.

Spoglio fumigation of persons, their apparel and their effects.

Introduction

Ralph Waldo Emerson, the American writer, suggested that 'Traveling is a fool's paradise'.[1] In normal times, few people would agree with that, but sometimes the analogy strikes home. Journeys by land and sea to remoter parts have always run the risk of bad accommodation, poor food, sickness, theft, piracy and civil commotion, while in the modern era, air travel may generate its own frustrations. None of these varied annoyances is or was entirely predictable, even though the risk might be high. This book, however, is about an annoyance which was known about, expected by all but the most naïve and virtually unavoidable even for the aristocracy. It occurred on the homeward journey, and the most seasoned adventurer was just as exposed to it as the diffident novice. The name of this annoyance was quarantine.

The term has become uncomfortably familiar of late with the spread of Covid-19. As our forebears learnt to live with quarantine as a permanent institution, we should be grateful, perhaps, that the practice has been so little used within living memory. Detention in past centuries was rooted in the fear of bubonic plague, which was endemic in the Near East. As other lethal diseases emerged, especially yellow fever and cholera, the rigmarole of quarantine was extended against them as well. Thus, it was a normal and unexceptionable hazard for any returning traveller until the latter part of the nineteenth century. In more recent times, shipping interests have worried about quarantine detention against SARS and the Marburg virus.

The paradox of quarantine is that the idea is so simple, but the ramifications are enormous. This is reflected in the literature on the subject, where historians have approached the concept from many angles. Most research has been under the banner of medical history, which has scrutinized the acrimonious and long-standing debate between the contagionists (who assumed that plague could only be spread by touch) and the anti-contagionists (who argued it was an airborne infection). Other research interests have focused on quarantine in a local context or on the material relics of the system, such as the frankings on disinfected mail. A recent study has looked at the constitutional history of quarantine in Great Britain, where it was part of the

DOI: 10.4324/9781003195733-1

royal prerogative and, therefore, controlled by the Privy Council, which at times was singularly ill-equipped to handle it.[2]

The same study also examined the commercial and economic implications of quarantine: when ships were lying idle for weeks at a time, often with their hatches open, cargoes were delayed, damaged or even ruined. Merchants and shipowners complained not only of their losses but of illogical and unnecessary detentions, which gave a mercantile advantage to other nations, notably the Dutch. But shipping interests elsewhere were no better off. In the seaports of continental Europe, quarantine was under the control of an autocratic board of health, independent of government. While this facilitated the workings, it brought allegations of brutality and commercial intrigue.

Aside from such medical, constitutional and mercantile issues, there is one remaining area of quarantine – arguably the most interesting – which has not been examined. This is the social cost of a system which brought so much inescapable and indiscriminate misery to individuals. Evidence of quarantine detention is not hard to find, especially in the nineteenth century when an appetite for travel coincided with a proliferation of publishers only too pleased to promulgate the journals of aristocratic and middle-class adventurers. But prior to that period, the number of first-hand reminiscences declines progressively, despite the existence of quarantine procedures from as early as the Italian Renaissance. There are good reasons for this: fewer people were travelling, the publishing profession was embryonic and quarantine restrictions were less comprehensive. It was not until the eighteenth century that purpose-built quarantine stations became usual, and well into the nineteenth before many countries found it politically or commercially advantageous to join in.

The present work examines the quarantine experiences of nearly 300 people, mainly from published primary sources. Reminiscences surviving only in manuscript form are difficult to trace but worth the effort. The evidence as a whole is sufficient for a balanced narrative of impediments to travel and an appraisal of the facilities (or sometimes the lack of them) which travellers encountered. Publications have been examined in English (from Britain and North America) and in French, as well as those in other languages, most frequently German, which have English translations. A researcher with wider linguistic skills could find more references, but they are unlikely to add significantly to these findings. This is because most information is based on a handful of quarantine stations in western Europe, especially Malta, Leghorn and Marseilles, and the recollections of one traveller echo very much those of another. Indeed, the information available about Malta is so extensive that there can be no aspect of the Maltese experience which is not recorded.

Although quarantine became a worldwide phenomenon, this study is largely focused on entry into Europe via the Mediterranean Basin, the Danube valley, the Caucasus and the Ottoman Empire. It pursues, in the case of the Mediterranean ports and the Danube, the main arteries of travel. Those brave enough to enter Europe overland from the Middle East and India encountered the rough-and-ready quarantines along the Caucasian border of Russia. As for the Ottoman Empire, it eventually introduced a system to catch those who were eastbound, a mirror image of western procedures, instituted at a time when some Christian countries were wondering whether quarantine should not be abandoned. The irony was that the West had always considered the Ottoman Empire as the very cradle of plague, chiefly because its view of the incidence and treatment of disease was fatalistic. Many travellers, both those returning from farther east and those visiting the Holy Land via the new and reliable steamer routes, were caught up in, and indeed caught out by, Turkish and Levantine quarantine.

Over three centuries there were undoubtedly quarantine stations which existed at one time or another which have not been examined in this book. Many were set up by Austria, later Austria-Hungary, along her extensive boundary with the Ottoman Empire; others were set up between Serbia and Turkey, for example on the river Morava. Most of these were mere encampments and seldom visited by the returning traveller. But purpose-built lazarettos did exist in Europe beyond the scope of those described here. At Toulon, for instance, there was a well-planned institution, but it acted as the military counterpart of the commercial lazaretto at Marseilles and is therefore outside the compass of social history. At Vigo, on the Spanish Atlantic coast, a lazaretto was built to act as the western equivalent of the Spanish-owned institution at Port Mahon, but it was irrelevant to the returning tourist as it was established later and not on a recognized route.

Some quarantine stations were introduced solely for yellow fever and cholera morbus, especially the latter. The threat from cholera was deemed so severe that every major port and border crossing along the length and breadth of Europe became an ad hoc detention centre for travellers in the mid-nineteenth century. Sometimes, as in the Baltic, it was a question of staying aboard ship; at other times, for instance at Rotterdam, it was a matter of staying aboard for a while and then going ashore. Occasionally, as on the Riviera between France and Italy, some old fort or port installation was rushed into use as a temporary lazaretto. Although references to detentions for cholera are relatively common, the quarantine stations were usually makeshift and discarded as quickly as they were introduced. They do not, therefore, appear in the Gazetteer of this study.

Britain also falls outside the scope of this work, for two reasons. First, there was never any lazaretto on anything like the scale or permanence of those abroad. True, some buildings were constructed at Stangate Creek in the Medway Estuary at the end of the eighteenth century, but they were dismantled for complicated reasons within the following 20 years. No reminiscences of detention there have been traced and little evidence remains on the ground. Smaller institutions in Scotland, such as the lazaretto at Inverkeithing, were underused and have disappeared without trace. Secondly, the quarantine facilities in Britain were geared more for the airing of cargoes, because most travellers returning from the East had already endured a quarantine before reaching home waters. That position altered slightly in the late nineteenth century when fast steamers imported cases of yellow fever from North America and the West Indies.

As I reread this work (drafted over ten years ago) during the Covid-19 pandemic, it strikes me that the perception of *noli me tangere* which underpinned the historical application of quarantine has not changed as much as I thought. Modern recommendations around touching and hand-washing are uncomfortable reminders of a literal doctrine of contagion supposedly laid to rest by physicians and parliamentarians in the late nineteenth century.

John Booker
Exeter, 2021

Notes

1 Emerson, R.W., *Essays: Self-Reliance* (1841), para. 41.
2 Booker (2007).

1 Reasons, regimes and routes

From the Renaissance until the middle of the nineteenth century, travellers returning to Christendom from the Near East were liable to a disagreeable detention to establish whether or not they bore symptoms of bubonic plague, which was endemic in the Levant.[1] The detention also allowed time for such symptoms, if any, to develop. The rationale for this quarantine was based squarely on the conviction that bubonic plague, that is to say plague characterized by buboes or swellings, was contagious. The boundary between infection and contagion was to some extent blurred (even when knowledge of the Latin roots of both words was widespread), but a contagious disease was deemed primarily to be spread by touch, while an infectious disease was airborne or waterborne. At the end of quarantine detention, a traveller was granted 'pratique', or freedom of movement.

In the Middle Ages, there had been no doubt that plague was contagious, and it was not until a severe outbreak attacked Marseilles in 1720 that any anti-contagionist lobby became significant. This movement was briefly encouraged by the illusion that the quarantine facilities at Marseilles were so strict and comprehensive that the plague which escaped from the ship must have been channelled by other means. Opponents of contagion argued that plague was spread by atmospheric conditions, including temperature and humidity, and the 'miasma' inhaled from foul smells. There was a degree of common ground with the contagionists, many of whom accepted that a polluted environment – summarized by the physician John Howard, in 1789, as 'putrid effluvia' – encouraged the spread of plague, if not its creation.[2] Both positions were to some extent justified. A century later it was discovered that plague was passed by the bite of infected fleas living on rats, so it was neither infectious nor contagious in the literal sense of those terms. But if the anti-contagionists were correct in asserting that plague was not passed by casual touch, it was also true that, if sufferers were efficiently quarantined, an outbreak could be contained.

Grisly epidemics in Messina (1743) and Malta (1813), when added to the infamous ravage of Marseilles just mentioned, ensured that bubonic plague was always the most dreaded disease. But in the nineteenth century came two other fearsome scourges. The earlier was yellow fever, originally

DOI: 10.4324/9781003195733-2

thought to be confined to the West Indies. But when a virulent epidemic spread through southern Iberia in 1803, medical opinion – although divided as usual – concluded that the disease had arrived nearer to home. Quarantine was used against it, not with any confidence but because no other defence was available. From the same negative reasoning, quarantine was used later against the second killer disease, which was cholera morbus, of which the first pandemic was in the 1830s. This was a far greater threat than yellow fever and caused many more deaths. But the disease was quickly understood, and sanitary improvements in urban slums were soon recognized as more effective in stopping the spread than quarantine could ever be.

Nevertheless, cholera affected quarantine in three ways. First, it meant that detentions (useless though they were) became as common on a west-to-east journey in western Europe as they were on an east-to-west. Secondly, as the disease became ubiquitous it was impossible to forecast the next point of attack, so that detentions were established on inland boundaries and indeed between one part of a country and another, where they had never existed for plague. And thirdly, it gave Turkey and the Mediterranean lands which it dominated (notably Egypt and Syria) a reason to establish quarantine stations against western Europe. This is a significant point because it underlines the religious differences between East and West. Christendom had traditionally been dismayed by the fatalistic doctrine in Muslim countries which would not allow the prevention of plague or even its treatment. Some western commentators wondered why the religious scruples of the Ottoman Empire which had prevented quarantine against the plague did not also apply to cholera.

Sultan Mahmud II asked Britain in 1831 for plans of a quarantine station which might be built in Turkey on European principles.[3] The British in London, who had no idea how a lazaretto worked, asked the governor of colonial Malta to arrange the necessary briefing as the island had a long tradition of quarantine and a good reputation among travellers. This intervention went well initially, but it was another four or five years before buildings appeared on the shores of the Dardanelles and the Bosphorus, after which they proliferated. Dr John Davy, writing in 1842, noted 50 Turkish quarantine stations staffed by Turkish directors and European doctors and mostly unfit for their purpose.[4]

The earliest quarantine measures anywhere are thought to have arisen at Venice in 1348. These were against arrivals from Turkey, and they were enhanced in 1423. But in the Turkey trade, Venice was soon eclipsed by Livorno (Leghorn in English), while the French finance minister, Jean-Baptiste Colbert, made Marseilles a compulsory quarantine port in the late seventeenth century for the burgeoning trade of France with the Levant. Thereafter, Marseilles and Leghorn maintained the leadership of the quarantine ports, vying with each other to dominate a clique in which Genoa, Ancona, Malta, Messina and later Trieste were also significant players. These ports corresponded with each other, swapping facts, intelligence and rumours about outbreaks of disease at home and abroad and administering their rules with precision and severity.[5]

As time passed, most ports of the northern or Christian shores of the Mediterranean had some kind of quarantine provision. They were anxious to avoid censure from the larger ports, especially Marseilles, if they were perceived as a weak link in the international defences. The penalty for too lax an administration was a punitive delay for ships from the 'guilty' ports arriving in the harbours of the clique. The apparatus of quarantine was often continued simply because ports were too timid to abolish it. William Baxter noted in 1849:

> 'We are aware that the reason assigned for continuing the quarantine at Malta is, that were it abolished there, Naples, France, Tuscany, and other powers would place all ships arriving from that island on the same footing as ships from the Levant.'[6]

To understand this better and to appreciate what the traveller was up against, it must be explained how quarantine was controlled. The organization in continental Europe differed markedly from that in Britain. There were also differences between countries within the mainland, but these were minor compared with the features they had in common. Policy ultimately stemmed from the king, grand duke, senate or other parliament in which the port was located, but the involvement of these higher echelons was nominal. In practice, quarantine was run by a local board of health composed of magistrates and merchants (not doctors) to whom the delegation of powers was absolute. The unaccountability of these bodies and the brutality of their code were shocking to travellers from Britain, where restrictions were haphazard and unpredictable, and most transgressions were met with no more than a fine. In Europe, offenders against quarantine could be summarily executed.

Against the simplistic continental practice, maritime quarantine in Britain was uniquely complicated. Impinging upon trade and foreign policy, it fell under the prerogative of the Crown, which exercised control through the Privy Council. Impositions of quarantine were brief, responding to epidemics on the continent which were generalized as 'plague'. Some comfort was derived from the country's island status, but during the reign of Queen Anne, any complacency vanished. Britain was subjected to a sustained risk of bubonic plague arriving from the Baltic, where it had spread rapidly from eastern Europe in a murderous and inexorable march. The prudent Anne took the issue of quarantine to the House of Commons to have her powers strengthened, clarified and confirmed. The resulting act, passed in 1710, was the first in a long series of quarantine statutes by which the power of the Crown was very slowly eroded, although it was not until 1753 that quarantine regulations became permanent.[7] The dichotomy of control between monarchy and Parliament and the resulting bureaucratic confusion had no parallel elsewhere in Europe. This British idiosyncrasy deserves to be understood but plays an insignificant role in the anecdotes to unfold, because most travellers had performed their quarantine before they got here. From 1896, quarantine in Britain was superseded by medical inspection arranged by port sanitary authorities and so became an institution of last resort. The rest of the world followed in a disjointed manner.

The imposition of quarantine between nations had usually been, to some extent, tactical and political. John Bowring, a well-travelled politician and businessman, wrote in 1838 that,

> 'Quarantine Establishments are, for the most part . . . terrible instruments of diplomacy and state policy. Under the plea of a regard for the public health, all letters are opened – all travellers are arrested and imprisoned – all commodities are subject to regulations the most unintelligible, costly and vexatious.'[8]

In the House of Commons, he singled out Russia for criticism, describing its quarantine officials as 'political functionaries', and he was by no means alone in his allegations.[9] James Minet was scornful of Russian quarantine near the Black Sea, ostensibly 'for the convenience of commerce', dismissing the Russians as 'deep designing thieves'.[10] Indeed, they were widely condemned for political quarantine along hundreds of miles of the north bank of the Danube. The Russian quarantines on the river Pruth imposed detention from west to east and were blamed on a wish to prevent 'the subjects of more liberal governments' from mixing with the locals.[11] Charles Terry put the allegation more graphically, claiming that the Russians wished to keep out not the bodily plague and physical distempers but 'the plague of knowledge'.[12]

If westerners approached Russia from any direction except the Baltic Sea, quarantine was always a problem. This was of no great consequence as relatively few travellers wished to go there anyway, and those who had experienced the quarantines on the River Pruth between Moldavia and Bessarabia or on the River Aras between Persia and Georgia were unlikely to visit them again. But the Black Sea port of Odessa was an exception. It was strategically sited, and its lazaretto, over the years, imprisoned scores of western travellers ranging from the adventurous tourist to Lord Durham, who was heading for St Petersburg as the new British Ambassador. At all other Russian quarantine stations the assumption, if not the demonstrable truth, was that detention was largely political. At Odessa that was not the case, and the quarantine there was planned to correspond with the most cautious practice in western Europe. This was in contrast to the attitude at Constantinople from which the Russian port derived much of its trade.

But Russia was by no means the only state to manipulate quarantine for its own ends. Political quarantine was a bugbear along the whole length of the Danube, where Austria was as much at fault as Russia. Furthermore,

Sicily and southern Italy were often biased against British shipping for complicated historical reasons, compounded by commercial jealousies. The Kingdom of Naples was particularly fickle. In 1828, the 1st Duke of Buckingham and Chandos, cruising the Mediterranean for his pleasure, was quarantined in Naples Bay having arrived from Pantelleria. Although that island was in free pratique with the mainland of Italy, he was prevented from landing. After persistent protests, officials claimed they had confused Pantelleria with Lampedusa, but Buckingham was scornful of this excuse: as Lampedusa was uninhabited, there was no need to hold it in quarantine at all. Gradually the truth became apparent. There had been an insurrection in Naples and Calabria with some 800 arrests, and the frightened King had already spent two nights aboard a frigate in Naples Bay. So the real fear was that Buckingham was arriving to orchestrate the troubles. He wrote in his diary, 'I really believe they fancy I want to become king of Naples'.[13]

Perhaps the most nonsensical quarantines were those between Egypt and Syria. Both countries were within the Ottoman Empire, but Ibrahim Pasha, son of Mehemet Ali the ruler of Egypt, invaded Syria in 1831 when his father fell out with the Porte, or Turkish government. Ibrahim won many battles and, despite his unpopularity, stayed in Syria until 1841 when he was finally ousted after the intervention of western powers. These machinations caused havoc in the 1830s for travellers arriving from ports such as Beirut at Alexandria, where they were detained without logic as the plague was endemic in Egypt. The true motive was to spite the Syrians for their unrest. In the 1840s, the tit-for-tat quarantine affected ships from Alexandria to Beirut to the dismay and disgust of many travellers. Unfortunately, it was uncomfortable for the British to sound too upset. A quarantine of ten days at Beirut against Alexandria was continued at the suggestion of Richard Wood, British Consul at Damascus, whose motive was simply to keep out the French. Their warships were steaming in sight of shore as France sought to match the local influence of Britain and Austria. For this underhand move, John Bowring saw to it that Consul Wood was exposed to the censure of the House of Commons.[14]

It was best for a returning traveller (especially if coming from India) to make for Alexandria to negotiate an onward passage. The port was so busy that the returnee, particularly if British or French, could normally board a merchantman of his or her own nationality. In periods of plague, however, which were frequent in Egypt, it was best to leave the port on the first available ship heading west. This vessel might well carry a foul bill of health, but it was better to endure an extended time in quarantine than run the risk of staying on in Alexandria. Having said that, the incidence of plague among Franks (as westerners were called in the Levant) was far lower than among the locals.

The next landfall was usually Malta, which a sailing ship could reach in as few as 16 days or as many as 28. An alternative route (not generally for the British) was from Alexandria to Marseilles, on which a journey time of

25 days was recorded in 1701, although in bad weather it might take twice as long. Both destinations were noted for their quarantine facilities. If no ship was available for Malta or France, the traveller could embark at Alexandria for Cyprus and take another vessel from there to the West. Cyprus was also a staging point if the traveller departed from Scanderoon, also known as Alexandretta, in Syria. This was the port for Aleppo and handled much of the trade of the Levant Company, the British body chartered since Tudor times to do business with the Ottoman Empire. Scanderoon is now the Turkish city of Iskenderun. The other port favoured by the Levant Company was Smyrna (now Izmir) in Turkey, and from there the route was also via Cyprus. Their fast, armed merchantmen did not call at Malta and would often attempt the long run to Gibraltar without stopping. If they needed to break the journey, they chose Port Mahon in Minorca. But ships of other nationalities did call at Malta from Smyrna, and the sailing time was around 38 days.

If no ship could be found in Alexandria bound for England, France or Cyprus, the traveller could make for Leghorn. This free port was the main entrepôt for trade between the Levant and the West and trans-shipped many cargoes destined for England. The lazarettos there were focused on merchandise, although many travellers were detained within their walls after a probationary period aboard ship in the harbour. Leghorn was also a destination for those returning from Turkey, but the voyage was not necessarily direct. An alternative route, especially from Constantinople, was to the Greek island of Syra, now known as Syros, part of the Cyclades, where the quarantine station had mixed reviews. This lazaretto only arose after Greek independence, and although Greece established other quarantine stations, notably at Aegina, Syra remained pre-eminent. Despite these precautions, Greece was never quite trusted by countries further west, and most travellers returning from there underwent another quarantine at Malta. An alternative sea route from Greece involved a short voyage from Patras to the Ionian Islands, which were under British control from 1814. Quarantine could be undertaken there or more probably at a port in the heel of Italy. In earlier years, however, the western traveller would have made for Venice, sometimes via the lazaretto at Spalatro (now Split), although the popularity of Venice for quarantine slumped in proportion to the weakening of its trade. From the early nineteenth century, the Austrian port of Trieste was the major quarantine station in the Adriatic, and it had the advantage of up-to-date facilities.

The traveller returning from Mesopotamia, Persia or land-locked Asia had a greater choice of routes. The most obvious journey was along the caravan trail beginning at Basra, reaching the sea at Scanderoon via Aleppo. But more intrepid souls travelled out of Persia across the Caucasus and thereby into Russia. The quarantine stations at these outposts were primitive, having little in common with those in the West, and lazarettos were rare. The traveller usually spent the night in a tent or under some old ruin, and sometimes in the open air. Once quarantine on these frontiers had been passed, the returnee had another choice – to continue overland through southern Russia or make for the Black Sea ports of Odessa or Trebizond where a ship could be boarded for Constantinople. Throughout southern Russia, the traveller would do well to escape further inconvenience and expense from quarantine procedures which were inflicted at stage after stage.

The Danube was another artery of communication. It is difficult to exaggerate the strategic and commercial importance of this river since Roman times, and in the nineteenth century it became a route of tourism in both directions. This relatively late popularity for leisure purposes was partly due to the political tensions along the lower river, but it had more to do with the geographical obstacles to the east of the Austrian border. It was not until the era of steam power that these were satisfactorily overcome. Even then the route from Vienna to the Black Sea was interrupted by dangerous rapids and the awesome gorge called the Iron Gate. At one set of rapids, a passenger boat capsized in 1839, drowning eight people in the cabin, which caused morbid curiosity in later years. The passage upstream through the Iron Gate was only accomplished by transfer 'to a flat-bottomed barge, with a very rattletrap gear and covering of wood, leaking considerably, and causing no little wonder in our minds how so fragile a contrivance could withstand the fearful rapids we were destined to pass'.[15] It was no wonder that some passengers preferred to walk up the towpath. The barges were then hauled through the rapids by men and oxen.

One attraction for travellers returning upstream was that the quarantines were generally shorter than those in the seaports. But when the Mediterranean lazarettos became more liberal in the late 1840s, the route via the Danube lost some of its appeal. In 1845, for instance, Robert Heywood at Constantinople decided to return by sea via Trieste, having heard 'such bad accounts of the Danube and the uncertainty of its navigation'.[16] The heyday of Danube travel was in the 1830s, when James Best noted with enthusiasm that the quarantine from Constantinople to Vienna by the Danube was only ten days, whereas it was 23 by sea via Syra and Trieste.[17] But whichever direction the traveller took, it was impossible to avoid several changes of steamer. Ida Pfeiffer, eastbound from Vienna, was directed into new boats at Pesth and again at Drenkova. The latter place was no more than an inn and a barracks, but it marked the start of the rapids. Pfeiffer embarked here on a small sailing craft for the journey downstream, noting that travellers in the opposite direction left the river altogether for that stretch of danger and discomfort. When she reached Old Orsova, Pfeiffer changed craft again to descend the fearsome Iron Gate, although the buffeting lasted only 15 minutes. West of Widin, Pfeiffer embarked on another steamer which took her as far as Galatz, where she changed ship once more, and the steamer *Ferdinand* made the last leg into the Black Sea and then around the coast to Constantinople. In total, then, she had taken six ships, four of them steamers.[18]

Although there were few quarantine problems on the eastward journey, the traveller knew it was impossible to stray far from the boat without risking challenge and suspicion. The niceties of sanitary discrimination became evident at Semlin, the last Austrian river port on the right bank of the Danube. It was not unusual to visit Serbian Belgrade from there, as the city lay close by on the River Sava, a little south of its confluence with the Danube, and its 'aspect' according to Pfeiffer was 'exceedingly beautiful'.[19] But Serbia was then part of the Ottoman Empire, and the quarantine barrier was absolute. One of the first to record the excursion was the renowned adventurer and writer Alexander Kinglake, who was accompanied across the border in 1834 by a 'compromised' Austrian official who lived 'in a state of perpetual excommunication'.[20] The trick in Belgrade was to see and not touch or be touched, or else the visitor would be detained in Semlin lazaretto for 14 days on his or her return. Charles Elliott, the vicar of Godalming, was in Semlin a few years later: he made the same visit with two other Englishmen, escorted by three boatmen, two health officers and a customs official. These escorts

> 'were provided with long sticks; and, from the moment we set foot on Turkish soil to the time we left it, they formed a cordon round us, preventing communication with others by means of their extended bâtons, and ordering us to halt whenever a crowd, or any other cause, placed us in danger of contact.'[21]

But when there was a perceived risk of plague the excursions were cancelled. Another English clergyman, the Revd George Gleig, chaplain to the Royal Hospital at Chelsea, found in 1837 'that the custom once was, but that it existed no longer'.[22]

The last Austrian town on the left bank of the Danube was Old Orsova, and from there it was Wallachia, now part of Romania, that bordered the river to the north, with Turkish control remaining for the entire length of the south. Pfeiffer noted that for the remainder of the journey the traveller 'is looked upon as unclean, and may not go on shore without keeping quarantine'.[23] Nor was it possible to enter Austria from Wallachia without detention. Elliott noted that the reason was

> 'purely political. Since a spirit of liberalism prevails in that and the neighbouring principality of Moldavia, the Austrian government does not wish more communication than is inevitable to subsist between the subjects of those states and its own; therefore, the notorious unhealthiness of the climate is made a pretext to establish a quarantine.'[24]

That echoes the criticism, recounted earlier, of Russian quarantines on the river Pruth.

Political instability in the lower Danube accounted for many of the quarantines regardless of the medical risk. When Elliott, heading west, reached

Silistria on the right bank of the Danube, the fortress town had recently been ceded by Turkey to Russia:

> 'but such is the jealousy of the Russians, that they will not suffer the steamer to disembark her passengers; and they have established a quarantine, more political than sanitary, to which persons arriving from Wallachia, as well as from all parts of Bulgaria, must submit, before they can enter Silistria.'[25]

The entire eastern end of the Danube, particularly on its left or northern bank, was disputed territory. In 1828, the Russians crossed the River Pruth and took Moldavia in a war with the Turks. The Treaty of Adrianople in the following year allowed Russia to control Wallachia as well, and there was then no question of landing anywhere on the left bank of the Danube without delay and scrutiny. Moldavia had its own governor, but Elliott described him as 'the creature and the tool of Russia'.[26]

The experienced traveller Edmund Spencer thought much the same:

> 'we may regard the principalities of Moldavia and Wallachia as entirely subject to Russian control, since the entrance to these provinces is watched over by Russian vigilance, in the form of establishments for the preservation of the public health, a vigilance which we know never sleeps.'[27]

Indeed, that vigilance lasted for decades. James Skene, a long-standing resident of the Near East, had business at Bucharest in 1851, which meant leaving the westbound steamer at Widin and crossing the river to Calafat in Wallachia, where he was subjected to a searching quarantine. In conversation with the director, Skene suggested he might not be very busy, but the man replied in so many words that his espionage responsibilities, crudely based on a specious detention of travellers, were continuous and heavy. Ah! thought Skene, 'This was letting the cat out of the bag with a vengeance'.[28] Public health had nothing to do with it.

In summary, the descent of the lower Danube was only free of quarantine or other complications if the traveller stayed aboard. It was impossible to leave the steamer at, say, Galatz and then enter Russia to continue an overland journey, for instance to Odessa. This eastbound detention went down badly, as it had no historical basis and travellers over many decades, if not centuries, had expected quarantine only in the other direction. Indeed, there was no way of ascending the Danube until around 1852 without spending time in the lazarettos of Old Orsova or Semlin to acquire pratique for entry into Austria. But by then the attraction of the Danube for returning travellers was all but over. It had never been more than an expedient while the European powers bickered over the longevity of contagion. Once quarantine in the seaports was minimal and steamers became better equipped and more efficient, the route home to England via Gibraltar resumed its earlier importance.

Reference to steamers raises one of the accelerating factors in quarantine's decline. It was steam travel, and a newly won sovereignty for Greece, which encouraged and facilitated the exploration of the Levant in the mid-nineteenth century. Enthusiasm for the new technology ran well ahead of the ability to deliver it. There was a lobby on Malta for steam-powered links with Messina and Corfu as early as 1824.[29] A more realistic link with Marseilles was proposed in 1829, but it was another three years before regular routes were established. The Austrian Lloyd Company began operating steamers out of Trieste in 1836, and by the end of the decade, they had reached most corners of the Mediterranean and the Black Sea. French steamers, and initially the British, were run by the state. The French had ten ships of 160 horsepower on the route from Marseilles to the East, sailing three times a month. The ports of call were Genoa, Leghorn, Civitavecchia (for Rome), Naples, Malta and then Syra, where the routes deviated to Constantinople, Athens or Alexandria. These ships were lightly armed with a crew of 30, as well as three officers, two cooks, two waiters and a stewardess to cater for the ladies.[30] From Britain, by 1843, P & O steamers were leaving Southampton for Alexandria via Malta on the third of the month and for Constantinople via Malta, Syra and Smyrna on the 25th. The voyage time from Alexandria to Malta was now reduced to five days, and the cost was around £12.[31]

Travellers were more than happy with the new phenomenon as some journeys by sailing ship had been dire. In 1806, Nicholas Biddle returned from the Levant to Trieste on a Greek ship. His journal recorded, 'I have rarely passed 18 days more disagreeably. They are much the most barbarous Greeks I have ever seen'.[32] His own food ran out on the voyage, and the crew were loath to share their own food until he had paid for it. 'These men are impudent & beastly', he concluded. 'When we arrived [at Trieste] they refused to come to the Lazzaretto to be paid but would not let my things leave the vessel until they saw the money'.[33] Eleven years later, Dr Charles Meryon, who had been physician to Lady Hester Stanhope in Syria, paid 350 francs for a passage for himself and his Angora greyhound from Cyprus to Marseilles on a French brigantine. The ship was loaded with 600 bales of cotton, stored in the cabin as well as on the decks. Meryon found the Provençal crew superstitious, cruel and disgusting. They blamed him for bad weather on the grounds that a Protestant was not a proper Christian, so they were suffering divine retribution. When his back was turned, they beat his dog. The cabin was flea-ridden and the ship was nauseating.

> 'The Provencaux . . . spit . . . on every spot, so that I had not a single resting-place on the deck, nor could I go one step without the apprehension of brushing with my long dress the saliva that was scattered and conglobated in every direction.'[34]

As for the food, two lambs were taken on board at Cyprus and slaughtered on the voyage.

> 'On the first day the blood caught from the neck was fried, which looked like pieces of liver; but this I could not eat. Next the liver itself was fried or roasted, and the tripe done in *fricassé*, but so badly washed that it was impossible to touch it.'[35]

The last straw for Meryon was that he could barely communicate his views as the crew spoke only their patois. The quarantine point here is that a lazaretto which might appear irksome to one traveller could seem like blessed relief to another.

Charles Rochford Scott, an army officer who had been forced to go by merchant ship from Malta to Alexandria in 1833, rejoiced a few years later that steamers were running monthly on that route, 'which relieves travellers just now from the embarrassing choice of evils to which I was subjected'.[36] That choice had been between a brig carrying coal tar, stockfish and bar iron and a polacca overloaded with building stone. Count Joseph D'Estourmel wondered what Archimedes would think of a sea furrowed by galleys without oars and sails, mistresses of all the elements and taming with their fire the fickleness of wind and wave.[37] From the English aristocracy, Lord Londonderry acknowledged 'the superior certainty of steam-navigation over sailing', enabling you to 'calculate your proceedings, despite the uncertainty of winds, calms, and sails; and this is very agreeable to those who have a distaste and horror of the sea'.[38] Phobias aside, Londonderry raised the strategic point that the essence of steam travel was predictability. Services could run to a timetable which only the most severe weather disrupted. Journey times were precisely calculated: for instance, 21 hours from Marseilles to Genoa, then nine hours to Leghorn or 13 to Civitavecchia, another 13 to Naples, and so on.[39]

Guidebooks, prevalent from the 1840s, gave advice to travellers intending to visit the Levant about the itinerary which quarantine least affected. Unfortunately, the steamer routes were so complicated and quarantine was so fickle that the advice was not always consistent. The experienced and authoritative Eliot Warburton advised those making for Egypt to begin at Greece and proceed via Constantinople, Smyrna and Syria.[40] There were no quarantines in that direction as far as the Syrian frontier with Egypt, and any which were imposed at that final border could be avoided by crossing the desert after leaving Jerusalem. The only quarantine to be incurred would therefore be in a western lazaretto, such as Malta. But T.H. Usborne advised travelling in the opposite direction. Go to Egypt first, he explained, and then take an Austrian steamer to Beirut; from there, sail to Smyrna and Constantinople. There would then be 12 days of quarantine at Syra on the return leg, but that would put the traveller in pratique for Greece. He or she could then take a steamer from Patras to Corfu and return via Trieste (with a short quarantine) or via Malta, where the quarantine would be eight days unless the traveller chose not to land.[41] Sir Gardner Wilkinson broadly agreed with Usborne, stating, 'Greece should therefore be visited *after* Turkey, unless they [i.e. Levant tourists] intend going home by the Danube'.[42]

It was evident that if steamers were subjected to the capricious and politically motivated quarantines which had detained sailing ships, then the schedules would never work. The British, French and Austrian governments came to the view, albeit painfully, that there should be an international conference to discuss quarantine and whether indeed plague was contagious. The first of these conferences was held in Paris in 1851, the precursor of a long series held in many countries which signally failed to achieve a great deal. Some port authorities were slow to place steamers in permanent pratique, partly from the genuine fear of infection and partly because a too-lax regime might be seized upon by another country as an excuse, commercially motivated, for a punitive retaliation. In this respect, Malta was in a particularly delicate position as it was Marseilles which was regarded as the most reactionary quarantine port, and the Maltese did business there. The sanitary police of Marseilles were subjected to a long and biting rebuke from the French writer Marie-Henri Beyle, better known as Stendhal. What would be the point and the pleasure, asked Stendhal, in a six-week round cruise on a steamer if quarantine were unavoidable on return? What could be sillier and more counterproductive than a 30- to 40-day detention at Marseilles at the end of a ten-day steam from Constantinople?[43]

Conditions on some steamers, if better than those on merchantmen, were indifferent. Lord Londonderry travelled between Zante and Malta aboard the *City of Dublin*, which his wife called 'dirty'.[44] His lordship was more blunt, describing it as 'a most ill-conditioned and badly-found boat . . . wholly unfit for the service which she was destined to perform'.[45] The perception of comfort and safety is important because the favoured steamers attracted the most trade, which had some bearing on making certain lazarettos more popular than others. For most people, the French steamers were the worst, which made Marseilles an unpopular port for quarantine. It is true that Cuthbert Young, writing about his experiences in 1847, found them 'very spacious, and the officers communicative and obliging', but this view was uncommon.[46] The Beswick family, in 1840, referred to the officers as 'dirty [and] disgusting'.[47] Mary Carmichael, steaming from Malta to Syra on a French government steamer, found the captain

> 'a curious contrast in manner to his compatriots in general: frigid as winter at the North pole; dismal as London in a November fog; clad in a suit of most impenetrable buckram; an evident enemy to the social principle, and shunning all interchange of thought with those around him, as if an idea imparted was a diamond lost.'[48]

Mary was among the first-class passengers 'for whom the fat stewardess reserved her sweetest smiles, hoping, with gracious looks, winning ways (and large donations of hot water), to merit a handsome silvery acknowledgement at parting'.[49]

T.H. Usborne advised using Austrian steamers, which were 'handsomely fitted up' so 'the traveller . . . will experience a much greater degree of civility and attention than on board the French line'.[50] On the other hand, John Gadsby, a few years later, thought the Austrian steamers dirtier than the French, although he 'subsequently found them improved'.[51] One of Gadsby's complaints was that the Austrian crews were lazy. At Syra, where goods and baggage were routinely trans-shipped, he noted that the process took 44 hours, whereas he ventured, 'I am certain that half the number of Englishmen would have done the whole in five or six'.[52] Indeed, Lord Londonderry notwithstanding, the British steamers had by far the best press. Eliot Warburton recommended them before the French, even if it meant two or three days more at sea.[53] The Hon. William Fitzmaurice, on board the British steamer *Flamer*, found that 'such, indeed, were the comforts and luxuries of the vessel, that it was more like travelling in a drawing room',[54] while Mary Carmichael found the *Great Liverpool* decidedly better than the French ship she had recently experienced: 'The good order, cleanliness, and regularity prevailing in every department are highly and deservedly praised. Princely fare is provided for the passengers; and nothing can exceed the liberality of the arrangements on board'.[55]

The result of such opinions was that most travellers underwent their quarantine at Malta, the western hub of steamer routes, because they arrived there in the favoured British ships. Even if they were destined to proceed from there to Marseilles or to one of the Italian ports aboard a French government steamer, they would break the journey at Malta to remain as long as possible within a British environment. The Italians were resigned to losing much of their business to Malta, so that by the mid-nineteenth century Naples had abandoned the practice of granting pratique. It must have galled many proud Neapolitans 'that from the east the city . . . is to be entered only through the harbour of Malta'.[56] By 1835, steam had so altered the dynamics of travel that the quickest return route for travellers to England was no longer via Gibraltar but overland from Genoa, a port of call on the steamer route from Malta to Marseilles. And Marseilles was the best port for urgent mail from Malta to London, as the coach service from the Midi to the English Channel coast was significantly faster than the haul through the Bay of Biscay. As for the eastern Mediterranean, Syra became the equivalent of Malta in the West for the similar reason that it was difficult to avoid. Gadsby reported that, 'The Austrian steamers meet here, one coming from Trieste, by way of Athens, another from Smyrna, and another from Egypt. They then exchange goods and passengers, and each steamer returns to its own port'.[57] As the service from Smyrna had begun at Constantinople, the traveller from Turkey had little choice but to return via Syra. From Egypt the shortest route to the West was still on the Malta steamer, but the attractions of Syra were compelling. The Austrian steamers made it their business to make the connections to Trieste efficient.

Once detention at Marseilles and Trieste became only nominal, other places saw the relaxation as an excuse to drop altogether a medieval procedure which seemed totally at odds with the scientific spirit of the times. Along the Danube, from around 1850, the excuse for political quarantine could no longer be justified when the medical rationale was undermined. Charles Pridham could enter Semlin without quarantine from the East, showing that the Austrians were at last being reasonable. But it was on Malta where most travellers noticed the difference. In 1854, Catherine Tobin arrived in the Grand Harbour at Valletta from Greece and was met by friends 'with a boat ready to take us at once on shore'.[58] That would have been unthinkable a few years earlier, but it was no exception then. Herbert Hall arrived at Malta without quarantine in 1855, although it had not been abolished in Syra, his previous port of call. At a similar date, the Dunlop sisters reached Malta from Alexandria, and quarantine was not mentioned in their journal when they went on land.

But the Turks would not relent. Quarantine in the Levant continued to strengthen, while in the west it continued to diminish. The West was being repaid for the humiliation of the battle of Navarino in 1827, when a combined fleet of British, French and Russian warships defeated the navies of Turkey and Egypt. Some bizarre comments arose from short memories. *The Boy's Book of Modern Travel and Adventure*, published in 1859, had a chapter titled 'Eastern Customs – Performing Quarantine', with no suggestion in the lengthy description that the notion of quarantine had begun in the West or had ever been used there. In 1864, a Christian missionary in Turkey, the Revd Henry van Lennep, mused that 'the plague had existed 300 years at least before Turkey could be induced to try quarantines; and now that there is no plague she likes them so well that she can't give them up'. But it was so lax, he concluded, that it was of no consequence anyway. 'So much for quarantine regulations in this blessed elastic land!'[59]

The later cholera pandemics, unfortunately, brought relaxations in western Europe to an end. Quarantine was particularly fierce in the 1860s, not necessarily in places where it had existed before. Mark Twain was one of many Mediterranean tourists inconvenienced and exasperated by clumsy precautions which had little to do with the epidemiology of the problem. At any port in that decade, quarantine detention was a real threat and caught many unawares. The American John Ross Browne and his friend arrived at Lisbon on a steamer from Africa and were dismayed to find a quarantine of five days. 'Well, this might be pleasant enough for the cabin passengers', he protested, 'who had something to eat and beds to sleep in, but it was pretty hard on Powell and myself, whose last crust had disappeared the night before, and who had neither bed nor blankets'.[60]

In the cholera pandemic of the 1880s, quarantine appeared briefly at places which could have been visited at will in the intervening years. Again, the eastern ports such as Alexandria and Constantinople were the strictest, confirming the anomaly that the places which adopted quarantine last were the most reluctant to let it go. For most travellers, by then the whole rigmarole was bafflingly archaic and even mariners could be confused, as the anecdote of the yacht *Griffin* at Gibraltar reveals. In January 1881, she reached there from Falmouth and anchored at the new mole, unsure whether or not to fly a yellow flag.[61] A boat was sent ashore for instructions and returned with the message that they must 'wait for *product*'.[62] The next day, the yacht was given pratique with a slight rebuke from the captain of the port. Product? Pratique? By 1881 it was all too confusing for words.

Notes

Notes that follow referring to works in the bibliography are described minimally by the surname of the author. The name is followed by (a) the date of publication, included to avoid ambiguity as two authors may share the same name; (b) volume number, if applicable, in lower-case Roman numerals; and (c) the page number(s). In a few cases those numbers will be in Roman when the reference is to introductory material in the cited work. The term National Archive' refers to the UK repository at Kew.

1 In 1729 the Privy Council decreed that the Levant meant anywhere east of a line from Corfu to Cape Rusata (or Rozat) on the North African coast (National Archives, PC 2/90/327, 338, 341).
2 Howard (1791, 25).
3 National Archives of Malta, C1, pp. 37–9.
4 Davy (1842, ii, 453).
5 For a discussion of these points, see Booker (2007), passim.
6 Baxter (1850, 272–3).
7 For a table of Quarantine Acts affecting Britain, see Booker (2007, 579–81).
8 Bowring (1838, 11).
9 Hansard (1842, lxvi, 614).
10 Minet (1958, 351).
11 Elliott (1838, i, 224).
12 Terry (1848, 285).
13 Buckingham and Chandos (1862, ii, 147–8).
14 Hansard, loc. cit.
15 Best (1842, 314).
16 Heywood (1919, 49).
17 Best (1842, 324).
18 Pfeiffer (1852, 36), where she complained that so many changes 'cannot be reckoned among the pleasures of a trip down the Danube'.
19 Ibid., 24.
20 Kinglake (1844, 2).
21 Elliott (1838, i, 96).
22 Gleig (1839, iii, 279).
23 Pfeiffer (1852, 29).
24 Elliott (1838, i, 95).
25 Ibid., 184–5.

26 Ibid., 207.
27 Spencer (1838, ii, 199).
28 Skene (1853, i, 272).
29 National Archives, CO 158/3 [unpag.], 7 December 1824.
30 Holthaus (1844, 262), who also explains that the ships were three-masted.
31 Warburton (1845, ii, 432).
32 Biddle (1993, 206–7).
33 Ibid., 207.
34 Meryon (1846, iii, 419).
35 Ibid., 420.
36 Scott (1837, i, 4).
37 D'Estourmel (1844, ii, 524).
38 Vane (1842, ii, 83).
39 Stendhal (1932, ii, 399).
40 Warburton (1845, ii, 432).
41 Usborne (1840, 82).
42 Wilkinson (1843, i, 54).
43 Stendhal (1932, ii, 398).
44 Vane (1844, 194).
45 Vane (1842, ii, 80).
46 Young (1848, 442).
47 Beswick (1997, 34).
48 Montauban (1846, 15).
49 Ibid.
50 Usborne (1840, 15).
51 Gadsby (1880, 133).
52 Ibid., 132.
53 Warburton (1845, ii, 432).
54 Fitzmaurice (1834, 74).
55 Montauban (1846, 132).
56 Watson (1853, 65).
57 Gadsby (1880, 132).
58 Tobin (1855, 249).
59 Lennep (1870, i, 37).
60 Browne (1867, 306).
61 The yellow flag, first considered in 1753, was introduced by Britain in 1789 for vessels liable to quarantine.
62 Maxwell (1882, 9).

2 Quarantine

The social leveller

All major quarantine stations in continental Europe embraced a lazaretto which was, in the words of John Henry Newman, 'as like a prison as one pea to another'.[1] This was primarily a range of buildings for the airing of cargoes. The process required large, open-ended warehouses where the goods could be unpacked, exposed to the elements (except rain) supposedly to remove the impurities and then repacked into bales. In some ports these facilities were purpose-built, although not necessarily from the outset, while at others an old barracks or even a convent could be adapted for quarantine purposes. A few lazarettos in the Near East were merely tented encampments. The word itself derives from St Lazarus, the patron saint of lepers, through an Italian route. The spelling, therefore, is more correctly *lazzaretto*, but in most countries the second 'z' was omitted and in Britain the term was often shortened to lazaret. In this study, for consistency, the word will be spelt lazaretto, the variation most widely found in travellers' memoirs, whatever their nationality.

Detainees seldom allude to the airing of cargoes and were not allowed anywhere near the process. In the eyes of a Mediterranean board of health, passengers in a merchant ship were rather a nuisance, distracting from the principal function of cleansing or 'depurating' cargoes. It was from this practice that the authorities derived most of their income, so facilities for travellers were a secondary consideration. (This was not, however, the position along certain overland routes of eastern Europe where, in the absence of significant freight, people were the focus of restrictions.) If travellers did not allude to the process of airing, they were nevertheless in no doubt as to why it happened. It was a common understanding that all notorious outbreaks of plague could be traced back in the first instance to infected textiles. Physicians were in broad agreement that the fibrous nature of cotton and silk, in particular, made them susceptible to carry plague. Another aspect of that disease which contagionists feared was its smell. This was so powerful that a comparison was made with the stink of the civet cat.[2] Such a distinctive odour, it was argued, was not wholly intangible: it emitted minute particles which could embed themselves in fibrous material and stay there for an imponderable period, poised to break out and attack.

DOI: 10.4324/9781003195733-3

The duration of quarantine for passengers must be seen in the light of what was deemed necessary for cargoes, which depended on the bill of health of the ship. This document, issued by a consular official at the port of loading, gave details of the cargo and listed the crew and the passengers. A foul bill meant that plague was (or had recently been) afflicting the hinterland at the time of departure, not that the ship was necessarily infected. Travellers in the age of the Grand Tour carried passports, but no individual bills of health. That had not always been the case. The Spanish adventurer Pero Tafur, wandering through Italy between 1435 and 1439, arrived at Milan where no person could 'enter the city unless first . . . he obtains a certificate which establishes that he comes from a healthy country, uncontaminated by plague'.[3] The Englishman Fynes Moryson, travelling in 1596, was a little more precise: 'they that goe by land in Italy, must bring a Testimonie of Health called Boletino, before they can passe or converse'.[4] Apparently in Venetian inns, the words *Ricordati della bolletta* ('Remember your Bill of Health') were written above bedroom doors.[5] These documents were taken so seriously that when Dudley Carleton, the new English ambassador to Venice, arrived at the border without one in 1610, he was initially refused entry. The Doge smoothed matters over but mentioned in mild rebuke that 'all obey' the rules of the sanitary officials.[6]

A clean bill of health for a ship reduced, but certainly did not remove, the period of detention for passengers. Foul bills guaranteed the longest and most stringent isolation. The traditional period everywhere (which might readily be lengthened) was 40 days. This term was based on no scientific or empirical findings and was essentially a superstition resting on several Jewish and Christian precedents, such as the temptation of Jesus who fasted for 40 days and nights in the wilderness. Forty had a further significance in quarantine because that number of days had to elapse before most ships could leave Turkish ports with a clean bill of health following an outbreak of plague. The word quarantine derives from the Italian for forty, *quaranta*, harking back to the trading pre-eminence of Venice in the Middle Ages. Italian was the lingua franca among Mediterranean boards of health and the language for most passports. Ironically, the Italian expression to undergo quarantine became *far la contumacia*, but that phrase did not spread to other countries.

A ship with a foul bill might spend several months in quarantine if there had been a suspicious death on the voyage. It was felt better to be safe than sorry, and political jealousies or commercial tensions might add weeks of delay at the whim of a bad-tempered board. One medical reason for inconsistency was that no early consensus existed as to the time beyond which symptoms of plague could no longer develop. Only gradually did that period fall to 15 days, and then to eight in the 1830s. There was no exact correlation between the quarantine duration of the ship and its cargo and the period allotted to the passengers, although they were not unconnected. Nor was there an automatic link between the period for the passengers and that for the crew; the latter would generally stay on board unless there was a medical reason for their isolation on shore. The only comfort for a passenger was that a period of detention exceeding 40 days was most unlikely unless there was a plague death in the lazaretto during the period of his or her confinement.

As the nineteenth century progressed, a quarantine for the full 40 days became increasingly unusual for travellers as long as the ship carried a clean bill of health. Nevertheless, there were significant detentions at Syra against arrivals from Egypt and Turkey and at Malta against Beirut and Alexandria. But once the steamer routes were running properly, quarantine in the Mediterranean could be avoided. On Malta, as at Syra, passengers disembarked from the steamer of their arrival to connect immediately with another. For England, the ongoing link for packet boats was initially Falmouth, but in the steam age it moved to Southampton. The quarantine station known as the Motherbank was situated off Ryde and served both Southampton and Portsmouth. A traveller from Alexandria to England, who chose to go the whole way by sea (rather than overland between Genoa and Calais), had to wait only two or three days at Southampton for pratique.

Leniency was possible because in most European ports the days of quarantine for a ship were eventually deducted from the length of the voyage. This concession had already been won for warships, but not without a struggle. At Syra the deduction was extended to yachts, but as the quarantine there was relatively long in any case, the yachtsman was still entitled to grumble. By the late 1840s, quarantine for ships at Malta was down to only five days, including those of arrival and departure, and this had fallen to three by 1849. Even Marseilles, stung by the criticism of Stendhal and the exasperation of other nations, took a leap forward. In 1845 the quarantine there and at Leghorn was still around 25 days; four years later detention was all but abolished for a ship with a clean bill which had been more than eight days at sea and carried a physician. For passengers on such a ship, detention was notional. In this respect, Marseilles was struggling to keep up with Trieste, which threatened to remove even the small business in passenger traffic left to the French by the popularity of Malta. By 1845, Trieste was offering pratique within 24 hours of arrival for clean-bill ships from the Levant. The commercial reward for Trieste was that it became part of 'Waghorn's Route', the itinerary ostensibly devised by Thomas Fletcher Waghorn of Chatham for reducing the mail run from India to England from three months to around 40 days.[7]

Before travellers' impressions are analyzed, it will be as well to discuss who they were, in terms of gender, status or occupation, and what they might have been doing in the Mediterranean. The Grand Tour springs to mind as a provider of inmates for lazarettos, but it was little affected by quarantine. Typical itineraries involved only western Europe – say France, Switzerland, Italy and Germany – and were essentially overland. Thomas Nugent, in his four-volume book of 1749 short-titled *The Grand Tour* dealt with Venice, Leghorn and Ancona without mentioning quarantine at all, although by that date their lazarettos were well-developed. In fact the word lazaretto appears only once in his guidebook and then during the description of Messina, where the institution was 'very convenient' and sited on an island.[8] But this was parenthetic. Nugent did not envisage his readers being detained there as Sicily would only inflict quarantine on tourists if they approached from the Levant.

If some travellers were more adventurous than others, they were more likely to take a tour of Iberia, for example, than a journey towards the East. Christopher Hibbert has explained that the 'journey into Greece . . . had never been part of the traditional Grand Tour', and there were solid reasons for that.[9] Being under Ottoman control, the country lacked the bankers and merchants who might have oiled the wheels of the tourist's progress as they did in Paris or Frankfurt or Rome. There was little polite society, and there were no spa towns or assembly rooms such as existed further west. In the countryside there were brigands and a festering spirit of rebellion. In 1832, Greece finally rid itself of Turkish rule and only then, long after the traditional Grand Tour had petered out, was the country popular with travellers. A nominal system of quarantine had been introduced in 1829, but with no history or tradition of the process, the facilities in Greece and its islands were often thought inadequate.

In hindsight, Grand Tourists were lucky to get away with their quarantine immunity, despite the relatively safe countries which they tended to visit. Some anti-contagionists argued that unrestricted land travel made little sense. There were periods when ships from even western Mediterranean ports were quarantined on arrival in Britain because of rumoured or actual disease. Tourists could return from the same areas overland in a matter of days without quarantine, yet they travelled in carriages lined with silk and other fabrics which were no less 'susceptible' than the bales carried by a merchant ship which was, furthermore, several weeks in making the voyage. Tourists were all the more fortunate to escape because their heavy baggage with pillaged antiquities routinely travelled back by sea and could be quarantined with the vessel. Some returnees may have pondered going home by ship, if only to keep an eye on their effects, but the fear of interception by Barbary corsairs, with consequent robbery, kidnapping or even death, meant that very few tourists returned by sea from the Mediterranean except in a British man-of-war.

In later guidebooks, advice about quarantine for tourists was inconsistent. The most important commentator on European travel during the early years of Queen Victoria's reign was Mariana Starke, but she was not interested in quarantine or lazarettos. Even the 1839 edition of her guidebook *Travels in Europe, for the Use of Travellers on the Continent* has no information on the subject. This is surprising as cholera detentions by then were widespread, and she was practical enough to produce an appendix dealing with such potential problems as passports and money. In being helpful to that extent, Starke's works were a forerunner of the guidebooks of John Murray and Karl Baedeker. The latter was too late for the quarantine era, but Murray's books tackled the problem in depth. His earliest work to discuss quarantine was published in 1840 and dealt with both the general issue and the relative strengths and weaknesses of individual lazarettos in Malta, in Greece and on the Danube. Murray summarized quarantine as 'the greatest annoyance to which travellers in the East are exposed on their return to Europe' – and that was written when the position had much improved.[10] Centuries-old traditions were not to be swept aside overnight by pistons and boilers.

Of the diarists and letter writers quoted in this study, some 25 were women, which is around 8 per cent of the published evidence. This seems a small proportion, especially as many wives accompanied their husbands, and women were more assiduous than men in keeping a record. The number of unpublished accounts (not necessarily surviving) of quarantine cannot be known, but it is a safe conclusion that the proportion by women exceeded this miserable ratio. Women were at a disadvantage when it came to publication. This might well be ascribed to old-fashioned values, but there was also the question of why the journey was undertaken: quarantine appeared incidentally in the memoirs of men while the substance of their books reflected the official purpose or outcome of their travel. Often they journeyed as a delegate or researcher of government or were funded by some learned society, the Church or a commercial interest. Publication was a way of putting the mission to bed, and information about quarantine is the historian's bonus.

There are, however, instances where the reminiscences of wives run parallel with those of their husbands, giving fresh information or a new slant on some shared experience. Judith Montefiore, for instance, published her private journal of the visit she and her husband took to Egypt and Palestine, and this preceded by more than 50 years the edited text of the diaries of her husband. The memoirs of the Marchioness of Londonderry, describing a visit to Constantinople and Athens among other places, were published two years after those of the Marquess deliberately, it would appear, to add a new perspective to the journey. It is tantalizing, however, that the quarantine experiences of Lady Mary Wortley Montagu and of the equally redoubtable Lady Hester Stanhope are unrecorded, yet both must have known the system first-hand as much of their lives were spent in the Near East. As if to compensate for these losses, the fearless German traveller Ida Pfeiffer was meticulous in recording her quarantine tribulations in several countries and explaining how lazarettos were conducted.

Julia Pardoe, another inveterate traveller to the East, noted that when she was incarcerated in the lazaretto of Old Orsova on the Danube in 1836, she was only the second lady whom the director had ever lodged there – which led to a patronizing welcome.[11] While other unescorted ladies (for instance, Ida Pfeiffer) undoubtedly took the Danube route, it is rare in the history of quarantine to find western women in any lazarettos except the best known. Malta and Marseilles were thoroughly accustomed to the reception of both sexes, but the smaller and more remote quarantine stations, such as those on the Caucasian borders of Russia, probably never saw a western woman at all. At other quarantine stations, typically in the Levant, there were certainly female detainees, and in some numbers, but they were generally from distinct ethnic groups such as Jews and Armenians, or even Greek slaves, and the authorities made no effort to extend to them the courtesies to which educated women were entitled in the lazarettos of the West.

Among men it is possible to create divisions according to their vocation or the motive for their journey. The early victims of quarantine were adventurers like the fifteenth-century Spaniard Pero Tafur, the Englishman Fynes Moryson (1566–1630) and the Frenchman Paul Lucas (1664–1737), for whom travel was an end in itself. In later years, it became more usual to journey for some specific reason, not necessarily altruistic. Book titles such as *Diary of an Invalid*, *Notes of a Half-Pay in Search of Health*, or *Wanderings in Search of Health* are self-explanatory. These were round trips, but many instances of quarantine befell those who chose to return wholly or partly overland from Asia, typically from the Indian subcontinent. Thus, Bartholomew Plaisted, an officer in the East India Company, travelled home via Basra and Aleppo in 1750, and Thomas Howel, a doctor in the same service, made a similar journey via Armenia and Asia Minor in 1788. Members of the military did likewise, either returning from their deployment or touring more widely with state backing. William Wittman of the Royal Artillery, who was quarantined in Egypt at the turn of the eighteenth century, was surgeon to a British military mission assisting the Turks. Thirty years later, Captain Richard Wilbraham of the 7th Royal Fusiliers was coy about the 'particular service' which took him to Persia on official business, but he was quarantined in the Caucasus on the way back. Major-General Alexander Macintosh took advantage of his 'military tour' around the Black Sea to pass information to the Royal Geographical Society, of which he was a Fellow.

Naval officers had many encounters with quarantine while on duty in the Mediterranean or Black Sea. The treatment of warships is a complicated issue inappropriate for this study of the fortunes of private individuals, but it will be enlightening nonetheless to distinguish between military and civilian detention. It has been noted previously that men-of-war were generally able to deduct their sailing time from the period of quarantine. The British were sticklers for this concession and justified it on three grounds: firstly, men-of-war did not carry susceptible cargoes; secondly, their complement included a surgeon; and thirdly, discipline demanded that everything on board was clean and tidy. The Royal Navy, nevertheless, had to accept that detentions were sometimes inevitable. There was no question in the nineteenth century of an officer acting like the captain of HMS *Assistance*, a 56-gun frigate which visited Malta in 1675. When the health officers asked whether the ship carried a bill of health, the 'Captain told them that he had no bill but what was in his guns' mouths'.[12] Other problems for the navy centred on the courtesy of exchanging salutes by cannon fire when entering a foreign port. Usually it was the British who took offence when salutes were not returned, but in 1674 a British man-of-war was denied pratique at Zante until she had saluted the Venetian garrison.[13]

While compliance with local regulations became the official line, there were still naval officers who spoke their mind about boards of health. An entertaining example was Captain Adolphus Slade, later knighted and promoted to Vice-Admiral. Slade spent much of his career as a consultant to the Turkish navy and was also a memorable author. He philosophized about the practice of quarantine, which he thought illogical and over-rigid. His prejudice turned to rant when he learnt that captains of British warships visiting Italy were suspected of giving inaccurate facts. Slade was incredulous that boards of health believed the assertions of their own guardians, so as to 'take the word of such scum, before the united testimony of the officers of an English line-of-battle ship'.[14] He envisaged a scenario: a merchantman and an English frigate left Alexandria together and arrived at Messina before proceeding to Genoa. At Messina, the merchantman took on a health guardian who would swear that no contact was made with any vessel following departure. This was enough to backdate quarantine at Genoa to the day he boarded. The captain of the frigate, on the other hand, took no guardian and was given no concession despite swearing the same declaration. 'What a balance!' exclaimed Slade:

> 'on one side, we have the word of a captain of a frigate, backed, if requisite, by his officers; on the other, that of a Sicilian, who . . . would, if resembling the generality of his countrymen, sell his wife or daughter, much less his conscience, for five dollars, or less.'[15]

In the annals of quarantine, the military are outnumbered by men of the cloth. These included chaplains to the army and navy, but most travelling clergymen were affiliated only to their Church and motivated by evangelism and philanthropy. The Revd Dr Pinkerton travelled as agent to the British and Foreign Bible Society, while the Baptist Missionary Society dispatched Joshua Russell and a colleague to India and Ceylon, which led to quarantine at Trieste on the way home. Many missionaries, such as the Revd Dr Henry van Lennep, endured lazarettos in Turkey or the Near East, and other clergymen were quarantined after a pilgrimage to the Holy Land. The vicar of Walsall travelled from a fusion of religious and personal motives, as did the Canadian priest Léon Gingras. John Gadsby called himself a 'Biblical and Oriental Lecturer' and his travels extended over seven years, as did his experience of quarantine. Some Quakers were also seasoned travellers, such as the celebrated American Stephen Grellet and the equally renowned English philanthropist William Allen. The Revd Dr Joseph Wolff, an assiduous traveller when he was not ministering to his congregation near Langport in Somerset, journeyed abroad over two years to establish the fate of two English army officers who disappeared in Bokhara. This was a particularly dangerous venture, but clergymen were among the boldest travellers. Another altruistic priest was the American Samuel Woodruff, who sailed for the Levant in 1828 as 'Agent of the Greek Committee of the City of New York, for the distribution of provisions to the suffering inhabitants of Greece'.[16]

Among the rest, there were barristers and academics, journalists and diplomats, merchants and mercantile observers. The last-named included John Bowring, sent out by Palmerston to examine commercial relations with the Near East. Others had more obscure political missions, like Julius van Klaproth, described on his own title page as 'Aulic Counsellor to the Emperor of Russia', who travelled in the Caucasus and Georgia by government command. Many of these men were seasoned visitors to lazarettos, perhaps none more so than the Frenchman Eusèbe de Salle, who wrote while in Malta in 1839, '*Encore quelques voyages, et j'aurai complété ma douzaine de quarantaines*'.[17] But de Salle had been an interpreter and journeys abroad were his business. Most travellers caught by quarantine could identify more easily with his fellow countryman Viesse de Marmont, who lived for many years in Vienna in political exile. In 1834, he went to the Levant in order, as he put it, to add new interest to his life, increase his learning and satisfy the innate urge of mankind to push towards a new horizon.[18]

As the nineteenth century progressed, quarantine was inflicted on two new classes of tourist at different ends of the social scale. There arose a new medium of travel strictly for owners and invitees – the large, steam-powered yacht. For many years, private yachts had plied the Mediterranean under sail. Sir Grenville Temple set out from Naples in 1834 in the *Floridiana* schooner of Captain Roberts: 'a small vessel of fourteen tons, originally built at Genoa for Lord Byron'.[19] On another occasion, Temple was a guest on 'a beautiful cutter of seventy-two tons' called *Gossamer*, belonging to the soldiering dynasty of Eyre Coote.[20] The cutter rig was normal for smaller yachts and some could be far from comfortable. Captain James Best made tours in the Adriatic on the yacht of his friend Captain Cunynghame and recalled being weatherbound. 'It is certainly . . . far from agreeable', he wrote, 'to find oneself confined a close prisoner on board a very small cutter, and with hatches fastened down to endeavour to keep the very small cabin from becoming flooded'.[21] This imprisonment was his period of quarantine on returning from Albania to Corfu.

The Marchioness of Londonderry described a journey westward from Turkey aboard 'Mr. Bentinck's yacht' called *Dream*, in which they performed quarantine at Syra.[22] But that was in 1840, and by then most yachts were rigged as schooners and attached to the Royal Yacht Squadron based at Cowes. Some of these vessels were quite roomy. Lady Elizabeth Grosvenor narrated her voyage to the Mediterranean from Plymouth in 1840–41 on the chartered yacht *Dolphin*, crewed by a captain, mate, carpenter, ten sailors, a cook, cook's mate and steward.[23] Apart from the authoress, the passengers were Lord Grosvenor, soon to become Marquess of Westminster, and the four elder girls from among their 13 children. On this voyage and many similar ones undertaken by the wealthy or aristocratic, it was impossible to avoid quarantine at one port or another, or to at least fall foul of the sanitary police. As the century progressed, these yachts were fitted with auxiliary steam engines. The best-known example was perhaps the *Sunbeam*, owned by the parliamentarian Thomas Brassey. The several voyages of this yacht were related by his wife, Anna Brassey, and were popular Victorian reading. On one trip, departing from Cowes, the yacht carried seven guests, 11 servants, cooks and stewards, and a nautical crew of 20, including two engineers.[24]

One of the last great steam yachts was the *Griffin*, about which General Maxwell was so enthusiastic that he named his book *Griffin Ahoy! A Yacht Cruise to the Levant*. This vessel has been noted previously in the context of a quarantine at Gibraltar. Although such names as *Sunbeam*, and certainly *Griffin*, would have meant little to foreign port officials, at least there was no scope for a phonetic misunderstanding. Not so, however, for the name *Mischief* in the Black Sea. Captain Slade recounted the confusion of a Russian quarantine official: 'we were at Odessa in the *Mischief* yacht, and puzzled him exceedingly with the name, which he wrote down as *Miss Chief*, asking us at the same time if *Miss* did not signify *Mademoiselle*'.[25]

The travellers at the other end of the social scale were the *nouveau riche*, drawn from the lower middle classes who had made money through the City or high-street trading. They took advantage of the new steamers to visit exotic places in which their presence, even 20 years earlier, would have been unthinkable. To British consular staff they were something of a nuisance as they spoke no foreign languages and were easily imposed upon by knowing locals. In fact, there was resentment in diplomatic circles that much time was spent steering bewildered travellers through the pitfalls of a foreign city, including its lazarettos. Thomas Cook, the originator of organized tourism, famously crossed swords with the British vice-consul at La Spezia, who accused him of depositing around Europe 'the sweepings of our prison-houses'.[26]

Such language did more damage to diplomats than to Cook, but then the consular service was often supercilious in the steam age. F.A. Neale, late of the British consulate in Syria, scorned the arrival in Gaza's lazaretto of caravans comprising 'Mr. Noakes, a retired butcher, with Messrs. Jones, Smith, Stokes, and Brown (who were something in the soap and tallow line)'.[27] It bothered Neale in 1850 that only the British, or more specifically the English, caused the problems.

> 'Spanish grandees, Italian nobles, German barons, and Frenchmen, whose families had pedigrees more antediluvian than Noah, were wont to submit calmly to the rules and regulations of the establishment, and

> quitted it on an intimate footing of friendship with the authorities; but no sooner was the proximity of a caravan of Englishmen announced, than everyone was thrown into a state of excitement; and all the twenty soldiers, with their truculent lieutenant, were immediately drawn up in battle array.'[28]

This breakdown between the diplomatic service and the tourist was in contrast to the relationship between consuls and travellers in earlier years, which was respectful, harmonious and constructive. The good offices of British consuls or, failing them, of a local merchant to whom the traveller had a letter of introduction were often essential. For ships' masters, consuls were indispensable in another sense, in that they granted bills of health. The consuls best regarded by the wandering Briton were those in Egypt and on Zante. In 1700, when William Daniel arrived at Cairo from Mount Sinai 'poor and disconsolate', he found the town so beleaguered by plague that the Franks had fled the streets and lived behind bolted doors. But the English consul's family, after hesitation, agreed he should

> 'come into their house as I did into the world, naked; which I consented to, soon stripping myself of my habit (which I was the more willing to do, it being very miserable, not having any shoes or stockings); after which, washing myself with some water and vinegar, Consul Fleetwood furnished me with other clothes, and with a great deal of humanity entertained me . . . making me, at the most doleful time of death and sorrow, as welcome as possibly he could.'[29]

If few travellers encountered such a life-saving reception, many were more than willing to mention consular help in their memoirs. At Alexandria, Consul Lee was a regular favourite. Joseph Sherer arrived in the port from India in 1823, not as destitute as William Daniel, who was just mentioned, but equally inconvenienced by an urban epidemic:

> 'Mr. Lee, the consul, was cordially kind to us; he gave up his garden-house, in the suburbs, where we performed a tedious quarantine of nearly four weeks . . . our exercise and enjoyment limited to a few morning visits to Mr. Lee in his *parlour*, a mark of no common confidence; for in general, during the plague-season, the Europeans shut themselves in, and peep timidly at visitors through a square hole in a locked door, through which they receive everything, even to the cleaned shoe, (after it has undergone fumigation) with a long pair of tongs.'[30]

On Zante, it was Consul John Sargint who first won the thanks of British travellers. Richard Chandler, arriving at the island in 1766, learnt the quarantine procedure from Sargint, who later visited him in the lazaretto.[31] Samuel Evers reached Zante with a small group in 1779, and they decided to stop there if only to escape from the squalor of their ship, where some had fallen ill. He wrote a letter to Sargint (later published) soliciting help in entering the lazaretto and seeking to discount some bills of exchange drawn on Venice. An answer came within two hours and the consul sent over his son Peter, 'who made me a polite apology for his father's not attending, on account of his advanced years'.[32] When the group left the ship, the vice-consul Spiridion Foresti took them

> 'to a very good house opposite to the health-office, which he had interest enough to obtain for us, to remain in during our quarantine, the Lazaretto being very unhealthy, and in other respects unfit for any gentleman to live in.'[33]

Almost immediately, 'we were visited by the worthy old consul, his two sons, and the gentleman before-mentioned [Foresti]. All of whom offered us every service in their power'.[34] Despite some disappointment with the discount rate for bills on Venice, Evers remained grateful to Foresti not only for the supply of 'necessaries' in their detention but for his ability to engineer them a reduction in quarantine from 28 days to 12, following a negotiated bribe to health officials.[35]

Foresti succeeded Sargint and became an important figure (respected by Lord Nelson) whose intelligence reports and intimations of plague were read by the government in London and the Privy Council. As the preceding anecdote makes clear, Foresti knew enough of the corruption on Zante to play the system with safety, in the interests of his British visitors. John Morritt sailed to the island in 1795 from Greece and was alarmed at the prospect of 30 days' quarantine owing to reports of plague at Smyrna. He therefore planned to double back to the Morea as soon as possible and return to Zante at a more favourable time. But there was still a difficult period to pass as he was actually on Zante awaiting a crossing to Pyrgo.

> 'We got a boat . . . and, as we were detained by winds, Signor Foresti smuggled Stockdale and me into his house about ten at night, leaving our party on board. We lay *perdus* one day there, so saw little of Zante. The inside of his house made us amends, for we found it quite *à l'Européenne*, and lived like Christian people for the first time. Nothing can be more attentive and obliging than the master of it, who is a great friend of Frederic North's, and procured his consulship through the Duke of Leeds.'[36]

When Zante came under British control in the Napoleonic Wars, the corruption of the health board ceased immediately and with it the need for counter measures hardly less reputable. For British travellers, Foresti became a consul like any other. William Turner, arriving on the island in 1813, 'went ashore, where I was met by Mr. Foresti, who hospitably provided me with every comfort which the rigour of the quarantine permitted me to receive'.[37] In other words, it was an orthodox respect for the rules.

Other memoirs indicate that British consuls elsewhere were equally competent, but few individuals became as well known because the volume of travellers whom they encountered was small. Yet Consul Moore at Ancona won a footnote eulogy from William Mure;[38] Consul Young at Jerusalem let travellers pass their quarantine in tents in his garden;[39] Richard Wilkinson was invariably conscientious at Syra;[40] and John Dick was one of a succession of British consuls at Leghorn gratefully mentioned in dispatches. Indeed, Edward Ives published his correspondence with Consul Dick in 1758, revealing that the latter interceded with the captain of the lazaretto for good rooms, sent a servant to take orders for 'such necessaries as you may want', provided reading material, visited several times, and summed up his role with the words, 'you have only to command me, and make me as useful to you as possible'.[41]

This reliance on consular help was by no means a British phenomenon. French consuls were similarly of service to their countrymen, while Austrian consuls greeted Ida Pfeiffer at Galatz and Alexandria and helped her escape from Odessa when she found it 'as difficult to obtain leave to get out of the Russian territories as to get into them'.[42] In remoter parts, a traveller could look for diplomatic help even from representatives of other nations, and Joseph Wolff, in quarantine at Trebizond, recorded visits by English, Turkish and Russian consuls.[43] Such courtesies were especially useful for Americans. Because their country had few envoys in quarantine ports, foreign nationals might fulfil that role, and in 1828 it was a Frenchman called Eynard who was introduced to Samuel Woodruff as the American consul on Malta.[44]

To balance the panegyrics, it should be mentioned briefly that not all consuls were consistently applauded. Robert Heywood, irritated by quarantine delays at Constantinople in 1845, met the British consul and 'found him to be only an old woman who knew nothing, and I think had hardly read our letters'.[45] But Heywood was an example of the relatively late traveller who expected British diplomats to rescue him from any strategic inconvenience. It was rare indeed to find a consul who was completely incompetent and rarer still to meet a consummate rogue. Yet one had existed, ironically, on Zante where Sargint and Foresti became so distinguished. The nationality of this scoundrel was French. There can be no grounds for disbelieving the narrative of his fellow countryman Paul Lucas, who arrived at Zante in 1703 aboard a corsair vessel which had captured the merchantman on which he was sailing.[46] In fact, the corsair captain was a humane man and gave the French consul, named Toligan, money to provide for the quarantine accommodation of Lucas and a 5-year-old child in his care, as well as for their onward journey. But the consul appropriated the money for himself, failed to find them a new ship and sent them only black biscuits, rice and cheese for sustenance. Lucas maintained that the consul had a sideline profiting from shipwrecks and prizes and turned to the Spanish consul for support. He was sympathetic, but Toligan dissuaded him from positive aid, and the food for Lucas and the child eventually ran out. After 42 days they left the lazaretto more dead than alive, but Lucas had the eventual satisfaction of exposing the machinations of the consul in the published recital of his voyage.

A handful of travellers visited lazarettos voluntarily. For some, they were an object of local curiosity in the same way as a military or religious institution. For others, the guided tour was part of a programme of international research. The most persistent visitor was the philanthropist John Howard, whose reputation ensured him a constructive welcome in the Mediterranean basin. The precedent formed by his visit to the lazaretto on Zante was sufficient to allow an inspection of the same institution by Colonel Winterton and his nephews a few years later.[47] At Leghorn, a tour of the old and new lazarettos was almost *de rigueur* for those who wished to break away from the study of antiquities and broaden their understanding of contemporary foreign ways. When Princess Daschkaw (or Dashkova) arrived at Leghorn from Pisa in around 1780, her inspection of the new lazaretto was retold at some length in her memoirs. 'One of the objects which most attracted my attention at Leghorn', she wrote,

> 'was the new hospital for performing quarantine, built by the Grand Duke Leopold. I could not but admire the benevolent idea of such an establishment, but I was particularly struck with the order and regularity displayed throughout all its arrangements.'[48]

The princess had another motive for the visit, which was to send a plan and details of the lazaretto to her mistress, Catherine the Great, in the hope that something similar might be built in Russia.

The possibility of contagion was not enough to conquer the curiosity of lazaretto tourists. Princess Daschkaw had been accompanied in her visit by the director, who 'seemed somewhat surprised' at her interest, given the risk.[49] In fact, she had faith in her precautions, which amounted to sprinkling her clothes and handkerchiefs with vinegar and sniffing a bottle of spirits of camphor. But in these measures she was more wary than certain others both before her and after. The Swede Pierre Jean Grosley, visiting Leghorn in around 1764, had been unaware that there were two lazarettos and that the second one, as he called it, was for people who were suffering from plague or had caught it while in quarantine, so it was more a plague hospital than a detention centre. Grosley sauntered into the first courtyard, where the sentry was unaccountably absent. He then approached the second courtyard, where the sentry shouted at him and jumped up and down, wriggling like a man being tickled. Grosley pressed on, thinking the sentry was soft in the head, and offered to shake his hand. But this made the man even more agitated, so Grosley withdrew and thought no more about it until later that evening when he recounted the tale at a dinner party. The others guests were aghast at his naiveté, explaining that if he had merely touched the sentry or his box, he would have joined the plague sufferers in quarantine, and, if he had attempted to flee instead, the sentry would have opened fire. Shouldering his embarrassment, Grosley narrated his exploit as a cautionary tale for the unworldly.[50]

In the nineteenth century, the lazarettos at Leghorn were still attracting visitors, yet the dangers of a misunderstanding were no less real. Joseph Douglas Strutt joined a guided tour in 1820 but still put himself at risk. The small group was passing a room which the guide identified as the place for fumigating letters. There were two steps up to it and Strutt noticed 'some apparatus' within that he was keen to inspect. He had one foot on the first step and had raised the other to touch the second, when the horrified guide yanked him backwards. He later wrote home, 'two seconds more & there I must have stayed 6 weeks'.[51] He was, as he emphasized, very glad to get out of the place. It would seem that such scares and incidents soon persuaded the authorities at Leghorn to prohibit lazaretto tourism altogether. J.C. Fulchiron, who visited the port in 1838, thought the lazaretto was beautiful and well maintained and that every precaution was taken to prevent plague escaping from within. But he added that this was hearsay, because if you wished to inspect the building, you could only get out again when your quarantine was over.[52]

With the right connections, it was possible to visit the lazaretto at Marseilles, which was wary of nosy foreigners. This was the one institution which caused John Howard a problem – partly of his own making as he had offended the French in a pamphlet criticizing their treatment of convicts and prisoners-of-war.[53] When Lord Carmarthen, the British Foreign Secretary, failed to arrange his visit at a diplomatic level, Howard took the dangerous (but successful) step of going there anyway, posing as a curious doctor.[54] Another reason for the non-cooperation of Marseilles was its fear that the British would get ideas for developing their own trade with the Levant, once they understood how an efficient lazaretto could be run.[55] But the French mellowed over time. The Dutch traveller Henrica van Tets gave such a full description of the '*petite ville*' which existed within the walls that she could only have visited it during her tour around France in 1819.[56] And Stendhal, confessedly '*un touriste*', made a point of marching to the outer gate although by then he was '*tout tremblant*', and it is not clear whether his nerves allowed him to penetrate further or whether his extensive discourse on the quarantine system was gained only from questions asked at the door.[57]

Even some Danube lazarettos allowed a cautious inspection by tourists. John Paget found himself at Orsova in 1835. 'The quarantine establishment was nearly empty at the time . . . and we were shown over the whole of it'.[58] Paget liked what he saw, which contrasted with the experience of Lord Monson at nearby Semlin. On the way to that lazaretto in 1839, he bought 'some very fine grapes' but they were no omen for what came next. The visit was not thorough owing to the absence of a keyholder to 'one of the dens', but Monson saw enough to congratulate himself that he was not an inmate.[59] This was not an isolated instance of lazaretto tourism at Semlin, because the Revd G.R. Gleig succeeded in reaching the middle of the compound in 1837: 'We were conducted, as strangers freely are, through this open court, and we had an opportunity of looking from afar, on the victims of the sanitory [*sic*] code'.[60] Gleig refers to them as being locked in 'cages', which explains the 'dens' mentioned by Lord Monson.

The lazaretto at Odessa, never a favourite among detainees, was another unlikely destination for the inquisitive. It was characterized as 'one of the most curious features of the place, and . . . one to which the resident earliest conducts the stranger, whether the visit of the latter be for purposes of amusement or commerce'.[61] For Charles Henry Scott, a morning visit to the lazaretto in 1850 was indeed 'rather amusing', but he did not say why.[62] Inmates would have disagreed.

Notes

See general note as to references stated at the end of Chapter 1.

1 Newman and Mozley (1891, i, 312).
2 Mead (1720, 33).
3 Tafur (1926, 180).
4 Moryson (1907–8, ii, 75).
5 Bates (1911, 360).
6 *Calendar of State Papers Venetian*, xii, 1610–13 (London, 1905), 69.
7 The extent to which Waghorn, who has a statue at Chatham, was personally responsible for the new route has been challenged by Freda Hardcourt in the *Oxford Dictionary of National Biography*.
8 Nugent (1749, iii, 366).
9 Hibbert (1987, 219).
10 Murray (1840, x).
11 Pardoe (1854, 331).
12 Teonge (1927, 57).
13 Carré (1947–8, 897–8).
14 Slade (1854, 543).
15 Ibid., 543–4.
16 This description, in block capitals, is given on the title page of his published journal.
17 Salle (1840, ii, 268).
18 Marmont (1837, i, 1).
19 Temple (1836, i, 149).
20 Ibid., 4.
21 Best (1842, 45).
22 Vane (1844, 163–4).
23 Grosvenor (1842, i, 1).
24 Brassey (1880, 420).
25 Slade (1840, 303).
26 Cook (1870, 60).
27 Neale (1852, i, 18–19).
28 Ibid., 15–16.

29 Daniel (1949, 82–3).
30 Sherer (1825, 197).
31 Chandler (1817, ii, 335).
32 Evers (1784, 130–1).
33 Ibid., 132.
34 Ibid.
35 Ibid., 133–4.
36 Morritt (1914, 244).
37 Turner (1820, i, 100). For reference to a recent study of Foresti, see the Bibliography under Chessell.
38 Mure (1842, ii, 311).
39 Borrer (1845, 401).
40 cf. Slatter (1984, 76–7, 79).
41 Ives (1773, 393–4).
42 Pfeiffer (1852, 34, 220; 1851, 263).
43 Wolff (1848, 399).
44 Woodruff (1831, 45).
45 Heywood (1919, 43).
46 Lucas (1731, ii, 430–41), from which all of the following references are taken.
47 Wilkinson (1806, 416).
48 Daschkaw (1840, i, 239).
49 Ibid.
50 Grosley's original French text (London edition (1770), iv, 20) ends, '*Ceci soit dit pour l'instruction des Voyageurs que la curiosité portera dans ces dangereux asyles*'.
51 Birmingham City Archives, Galton MSS., 3101/C/E/2/1/2.
52 Fulchiron (1843, i, 5).
53 Gibson (1901, 135).
54 Ibid.; Booker (2007, 218).
55 Field (1855, 96–9).
56 Tets (1966, 145).
57 Stendhal (1932, ii, 401).
58 Paget (1839, ii, 125).
59 Monson (1840, 130).
60 Gleig (1839, iii, 277–8).
61 Brooks (1854, 29).
62 Scott (1854, 339).

3 First impressions

When a ship from the Levant arrived in a western seaport, it was intercepted before docking to establish the status of its bill of health. A foul-bill ship might be banished from the harbour if any sickness was reported aboard. Sometimes (as at Marseilles) there were convenient islands nearby where a vessel could be detained under a quarantine of observation. In the case of a clean bill (or indeed a foul bill which gave no cause for alarm), the ship docked or the master was escorted ashore to the bureau of health, known in some places as the pratique office or *sanita*, where he presented his papers. This office was often purpose built and on the quayside. Once the documentation had been taken by tongs, the master was then questioned about the circumstances of the voyage and sworn to the truth of his answers. The ship's bill of health, which included the names of all on board, was examined in more detail. If there was a discrepancy between the bill and the facts (for instance, if the ship had an extra person on board or, more alarmingly for the interrogators, a person missing), there had to be a very good reason. Passengers then left the ship to enter the lazaretto, although at Leghorn they remained on board for a probationary period. It was also possible to stay aboard at some other ports, but it usually reduced the period of detention to come ashore.

At this point it was often alleged that privileged people, especially the aristocracy, were treated more favourably. For boards of health the question was perennially difficult. The natural deference of past generations towards people of higher social rank or political importance sat awkwardly against the inclusiveness which quarantine demanded. All western lazarettos were at pains to deny favouritism on any grounds, because the penalty for being caught out would lead other ports to impose punitive quarantines against ships from the offending country. There was also the argument that, if governments really believed in quarantine, they would not put their own people at risk for the sake of politeness. Yet despite the dangers and denials, favouritism undoubtedly existed. John Bowring stated in the House of Commons in 1843 that 'all sanatory [*sic*] regulations are turned adrift when very great men are concerned', and in that allegation he was only repeating a popular conception.[1] In 1821, for

DOI: 10.4324/9781003195733-4

instance, Peter Laurent took the laxity of his arrival at Athens as a reason to postulate that 'members of government and people of distinction' frequently avoided quarantine, although they should know better by setting an example.[2]

An early instance of favoured treatment dates from 1605 when Baron de Beauvau arrived at Malta from the Levant. Grand Master de Vignancourt, despite the foul bill of health of the ship, had him received by the knights and taken to the palace for a reception '*avec toute sorte d'honneur*', after which the Baron was taken to special lodgings.[3] This was not exceptional as a Roman gentleman, Pietro della Valle, arriving in 1625 was allowed ashore to spend his quarantine in similar accommodation.[4] The courtesies he was extended never wavered, despite concern that Sicily might use the excuse of quarantine irregularity to stop exporting corn to Malta. And it was not only social rank which impressed the Maltese establishment before the days of French and then British control. When a ship arrived in the Grand Harbour from Smyrna in 1724, local gentlemen were so taken by the beauty of a lady passenger that presents, including wine and game, were sent out to the ship. The quarantine term was then halved for the husband and presumably the rest, '*par rapport à sa belle femme*'.[5]

Under British rule, the quarantine authorities on Malta were more circumspect. In fact, the importance of maintaining the island's trading links with Marseilles and Sicily led almost to paranoia on the part of the Maltese board of health, of which the governor was president. But concessions might still arise. Joseph Woods wrote cryptically from the Malta lazaretto in 1818 that, 'The governor . . . seems to use a dispensing power, which shows that he does not think the quarantine regulations of much importance'.[6] But successive governors granted dispensations very rarely. Judith Montefiore wrote that 'we were to receive the indulgence of seven or eight days' grace; but this was to be kept a secret, as persons are generally tenacious of preference being shown in these cases'.[7] In fact they had ten days' grace, 'a favour not usually obtained'.[8] When a governor interfered in later years, it was not to shorten the period of detention but usually to improve conditions. In 1840, Governor Bouverie intervened to secure 'the most comfortable quarters' in Fort Manoel for the Honourable Mary Damer and her party.[9] It would appear that Sir Walter Scott, visiting Malta in his frailty in 1831 and occupying 'the decayed chambers of a magnificent old Spanish palace', had received a similar concession from Governor Ponsonby, but the description of his lodgings is open to question.[10]

It will be recounted later that the children of Ambassador Rashid Pasha were allowed the privilege of boating from Malta lazaretto, but minors were so infrequent in lazarettos anywhere that an excuse for this indulgence can easily be made. And the British had support for their generally conscientious approach. The Persian Prince Najaf Koolee Meerza, doing quarantine at Malta on his way to England in 1836, thought the Maltese authorities a model of correctness:

> 'God protect! If any one should break the law of this place, or do any thing contrary to its regulation, though it should be the emperor of all the face of the earth, and offer millions of money, it would not be accepted; nor could he escape the punishment.'[11]

The experience of the Marquess and Marchioness of Londonderry, four years later, corroborated the Persian's impression, although at British-run Corfu they had experienced exactly the kind of concessions which they had no doubt been expecting. The Marquess, on their arrival from Greece, recalled being dismayed at the thought of detention in a 'very bad' Corfu lazaretto two miles off shore, but he need not have worried:

> 'Under the kind assistance . . . of the Lord High Commissioner, Sir H. Douglas, who showed me every possible care and attention, we prevailed on the quarantine captain, at the office of health, to give us two rooms of his own on shore; and the physician, who held the office of inspector of health, had, subsequently, the very great kindness to vacate his own lodgings, two really good rooms, with fire-places. In these four small apartments we were stowed away, ourselves and our servants, with no inconsiderable satisfaction. . . . Indeed, although we had eight weary days to pass in this imprisonment, I must say that as our friends from the yachts came and dined with us each day, as we had luxuries of all kinds sent from the governors, in viands, for the table; for the senses beautiful flowers, and for the mind quantities of books and newspapers, the time did not pass heavily nor disagreeably.'[12]

When the Marquess and Marchioness reached Malta a few weeks later, they suffered another quarantine as the Ionian Islands were seldom in pratique with ports further to the west, even if they were British-owned. But this time there was none of the subservience they were used to, and the Marchioness noted in her journal:

> 'we were transferred from this dirty vessel [the steamer *City of Dublin*] to the Lazzaretto . . . and in this dreary abode, with stone floors and stone walls, cut off from the rest of the world, we vegetated five whole days.'[13]

Dinner with the governor on their release was hardly enough to balance the indignity.

Despite the protestations of other quarantine ports that their rules were applied without fear or favour, only at Marseilles can that claim be believed.

Certainly, the board of health at Leghorn had a reputation for uncompromising behaviour, but at times it weakened. When Captain Sutherland (a soldier) arrived there from Greece in 1788, he had little to complain about:

> 'Lord Hervey, who has succeeded Sir Horace Mann, as Ambassador at Florence, happening to be at Leghorn, interested himself in our favor; in consequence of which, our quarantine was only fifteen days, and we got pratick [pratique] the day before yesterday.'[14]

He might well have been detained for twice that period. In 1814, the 6th Duke of Bedford and his entourage arrived at Leghorn from Algeciras, a journey which would not normally have involved quarantine. But Gibraltar, across the bay from the Spanish port, was suffering badly at that time from yellow fever, and the Duke was shocked to be given 40 days in the lazaretto at Leghorn. He appealed immediately, and 'on a representation being made to the Grand Duke, the Govr. reduced the Term of our Quarantine to 20 days'.[15]

Naples was another port which considered itself strict, and its inflexible and sometimes illogical stances annoyed both travellers and shipowners over centuries. But even Naples could be won over. When Sir Walter Scott and his companions reached the city in 1831, their quarantine was cut short by the King of Naples and they quickly established themselves in the Palazzo Caramanico.[16] Trieste was a better-run quarantine port, but it suffered agonies in the 1830s for showing an indulgence towards Lord Strangford. His lordship arrived there on a British frigate on his way to a congress in Vienna. When the 'courtesy' of his pratique leaked out, health authorities in Italy and Marseilles retaliated against Austrian shipping, 'and endless steps had to be taken before this burdensome measure was repealed at the end of nine or ten months'.[17] But despite some lapses, Trieste too was conscientious. When Thomas Howel arrived in 1788 on his way home from India, he and his friends were told they would be detained in the lazaretto for 42 days. As his group was in perfect health, they applied for a remission and the period was dropped to 35 days.[18] But this was still a significant detention as the original tariff was excessive. It was to be another 40 years before Trieste led the way to a more liberal regime in the Mediterranean as a whole.

In minor quarantine stations, where the opinion of other health boards was of little concern, it was usually possible to find a senior figure who could influence local officials or even overrule them. Barletta, in southern Italy, was an example. The Quaker missionary Stephen Grellet arrived there in 1819 and was grateful to have privacy:

> 'It is by the kind attention of General Maitland, who wrote, it appears on purpose, that they have given me these separate rooms; a very great accommodation; for in the other parts of the lazaretto they are much crowded, – men, women, and children of various colours and nations.'[19]

Alexander Kinglake had a similar experience at Barletta, where he was threatened with a quarantine of three weeks. He 'wrote immediately to our minister at Naples & he very kindly exerted himself to procure some remission of my imprisonment but was only able to gain for me three days – these however were precious'.[20] Elsewhere in Italy, Queen Caroline landed as close to Rome as possible in 1814, having shaken off the attention of a Barbary corsair.

> 'Her Majesty made an immediate application to the Pope, for his permission to land without performing quarantine. . . . The [affirmative] answer of his Holiness reached us . . . and we landed, full of gratitude for our escapes, and of anxiety for repose.'[21]

In quarantine stations further east, and in those of central Europe, concessions might be granted at the whim of the director. In 1806, Nicholas Biddle landed on the Ionian island of Ithaca, where the governor, being 'a clever young man from Venice . . . dispensed with the quarantine but gave me a guard by way of preserving the form'.[22] When the Duke of Ragusa arrived at Alexandria from Syria in 1834, he was refused pratique. When this news reached Mehemet Ali, who had already set out from Alexandria for Cairo, he doubled back to greet the visitor and put one of his own palaces on the seashore at the Duke's disposal. Nothing was neglected to make the Duke's quarantine agreeable, and the period was reduced to a token seven days. It became a talking point in Egypt that Mehemet Ali had never before been so obliging to a Frank.[23] Captain the Honourable George Keppel experienced favour farther east. In 1824 he was travelling north out of Persia towards Astrakhan, along the west shore of the Caspian Sea. 'At midnight', he recounted,

> 'I arrived at the Quarantine-house, where I heard I should be detained four days. I found here three Kizliar merchants, who had passed me [on the route]. . . . I wrote a letter to the Governor of Astrakhan in the morning, which brought me a release in the afternoon; but my three companions had to remain in confinement during the whole period.'[24]

Grace and favour aside, there were formalities at the entrance to every lazaretto. All papers that came from the ship, whether from the master or his passengers, were treated with suspicion – not for the content ostensibly but for latent infection. In some quarantine stations, notably on the Danube, the paperwork was 'duly fumigated in an adjoining room which is eternally smoking with the infallible antidote [to plague]', before being taken up in a pair of tongs for examination.[25] At Semlin, the 'eyes, nose and complexion of the traveller' were 'carefully delineated' by the officials, together with a record of 'birth, parentage and education', but few other health authorities bothered with such a rigmarole.[26] Then, in some lazarettos, it was the turn of the traveller to be purified. This was far from being a formality and produced vehement criticism of the quarantine process. Although fumigation was most normal at the beginning of the detention, it might also occur during and at the end.

People were subjected to a noxious compound of heated herbs and chemicals, which left them nauseated, choking and fearing suffocation. Ironically, the most harrowing experiences were in the East where the quarantine tradition was shortest. In many ports, especially Odessa, there was emphasis on the *spoglio*, a system whereby new arrivals stripped naked to be inspected and purified before changing into fresh clothes supplied either by local contacts or by the quarantine authorities. Their own clothes were returned after fumigation. Despite the Italian name, this practice was never widespread in the Christian Mediterranean lazarettos, although instances can be found, notably at Syra. An early reference to the process is in the memoirs of the diplomat Robert de Dreux, who returned to Toulon from the Levant in the middle of the seventeenth century. He and a Jesuit priest from his ship were spared the indignity of stripping with the crew. Instead, a health official escorted them to his nearby house where a fumigation chamber was rigged out in the garden and they could undress with modesty. The diplomat went in first and got out quickly just before the fumes became unbearable. The Jesuit had to enter just after him but was overcome immediately and tumbled out of the door on the verge of asphyxia.[27]

Russia adopted the *spoglio* in response to the plague threat from neighbouring Turkey. The necessity to strip naked in front of others went down badly with many people arriving at Odessa, especially the British. Captain Jesse 'ventured to object to this public display of my person' but was told that the rules were inflexible.[28] Some consolation to him was the opportunity to be smug when someone less presentable exposed himself: he was fascinated 'by the entrance of a naked Tartar, of hideous aspect; his deformed person was covered with burns and scars, and his whole appearance more like Quasimodo's, than any being, real or imaginary, I ever heard or read of'.[29] Adolphus Slade made a similar plea for modesty but was no more polite about the peculiarities of others. He wrote, 'I experienced, as an Englishman, a natural reluctance to submit to such exposure; nor was I reconciled to the idea by the assurances that Count Orloff, with other distinguished officers, and even Lord Durham, had done so'.[30] In fact, Slade was luckier than some, being 'permitted . . . to enter the inspection room first and alone'.[31] He then had a grandstand view of the rest of his group, who were granted no privileges. Slade disparaged the naked appearance of others, conniving with the quarantine doctor in gaiety and innuendo: 'a short fattish man' appeared to be the prototype for Mr. Pickwick, and a 'son of Levi' was the butt of a smutty reference to circumcision.[32] The only man to impress Slade was their soldier-guardian, 'a figure for a sculptor to have gazed on with pleasure. I never saw a finer specimen of well-set herculean strength'.[33]

Degrading as it was, the *spoglio* at Odessa had a funny side when people saw how ridiculous they appeared afterwards in their borrowed attire. Charles Terry

> 'could not forbear laughing, although tolerably disgusted with my strange dress: my under clothing was of a very rough and scanty character, my thin boots of an enormous size, my trousers big enough [for a giant] . . . their fashion and marks of use denoting their descent from a long past generation. . . . I was then roofed in with a thick cotton pyramidal night cap'.[34]

When Terry recovered his own clothes after their 48 hours of fumigation, he was surprised that they were not more damaged and discoloured.

Women were not exempt from the *spoglio* but were generally examined by another female. At Calorash on the Danube, they were inspected by a 'matron'.[35] This also happened normally at Odessa but, to the outrage of some British visitors, women there might also be examined by men. Adolphus Slade explained:

> 'Ladies are inspected by their own sex; that is sufficiently disagreeable, for the women employed imagine they are doing their duty by being very particular. At times even that attention to decorum is wanting. A few months before my visit to Odessa, two English ladies (one of whom was the wife of a clergyman) had to expose themselves to the director and surgeon. They remonstrated, as a matter of course; but their remonstrances were unheeded: the individuals in question insisted upon exercising their authority. I hope, for the credit of Russia, that this tale may be untrue.'[36]

Whether it was untrue or not, Slade's experiences occurred in 1838 when a more decorous procedure had been working for some time. Three years earlier, John Stephens, after his own examination, asked the doctor

> 'whether he held the same inquisition upon the fair sex; to which he replied with a melancholy upturning of the eyes, that in the good old days of Russian barbarism this had been part of his duties, but that the march of improvement had invaded his rights, and given this portion of his professional duties to a *sage femme* [midwife].'[37]

This was perhaps the profession of the formidable woman of whom Charles Terry heard an anecdote in 1846. He had entered quarantine at Odessa with, among others, a count and countess. Before the sexes were separated, a 'doctress' took the latter in hand and insisted she let down her long hair on the assumption it was false, 'envious perhaps herself, for she could only boast of a little severe top knot, and that made up of all that could be gathered together from all quarters of her uninteresting sour-faced head'.[38]

Another checkpoint to favour the *spoglio* was Taganrok on the Sea of Azov, where travellers stripped in marquees erected on the beach.[39] The practice spread to Alexandria where quarantine could be shortened for those undergoing an optional 'ordeal', in which 'the voyager strips off his clothes . . . which are taken and smoked; and having washed himself in a warm bath, he puts on other vestments, sent from the shore'.[40] A bath was not part of the compulsory Russian *spoglio*, but it was included in the process at Syra, which rewarded the volunteer with a reduction in quarantine of five days.[41] At Trieste, a similar system prevailed as late as 1840 when Francis Galton shortened his quarantine by 'three or four days' by swimming naked across a dock from one quay to the other. He had agreed with 'one of the old-clothes men' that he would sell him his existing apparel before jumping in and buy a new outfit from him when he climbed out.[42]

Even when the *spoglio* was not enforced, there were uncomfortable requests for nudity. John Stephens, undergoing medical inspection at Odessa in 1835, was one of a naked group that was ordered, as he explained, to 'slap our hands smartly under our arms and upon our groins, these being the places where the fatal plague-marks first exhibit themselves'.[43] Such precautions had long been intermittent in the West. At Otranto in southern Italy, in 1819, Peter Laurent suffered in a similar way: the physician 'ordered us to strike our armpits and hips, the spots where the plague-ulcers usually make their first appearance'.[44] Pierre de Saumery had encountered an unusual variant of this precaution at Leghorn in 1724. He was undergoing an initial quarantine on board the ship which brought him. After ten days, a doctor came alongside but kept his distance. Everyone had to strip '*nud comme la main*', and the doctor, sitting in his rowing boat, probed them for buboes with the end of a stick.[45] There was a similar requirement to strip at Messina around that time, but the practice was never widespread and eventually petered out. It is not clear what arrangements were made at these ports for the examination of women, rare as they were in the lazarettos of Messina and Otranto.

The same Pierre de Saumery had another bad experience at Leghorn where he was fumigated with burning sulphur and strong herbs for half an hour. The only way to avoid suffocation from '*ce maudit parfum*' was to lie face down on the stone slabs. He came out, he claimed, more dead than alive and as black as a chimney sweep.[46] At Marseilles in 1750, Bartholomew Plaisted found the ordeal much shorter than that at Leghorn, but the rigmarole was similar:

> 'They make a Straw Fire in the Middle of your Room, and throw on it a Mixture of several Drugs, and when the Room is full of Smoke, they oblige you to enter it, when the Door and Windows are shut. Here you must stay about four Minutes.'[47]

By 1807 the process at Marseilles had lengthened, and Stephen Grellet found himself in a fumigating chamber for about fifteen minutes. 'I had a small aperture to breathe through' he commented, 'else I should have been suffocated'.[48] Ida Pfeiffer found conditions no better at Alexandria in 1842, but the ordeal came later in her detention. After seven days all inmates were sent to their rooms in the early morning.

> 'Doors and windows were then locked, and great chafing-dishes were brought, and a dreadful odour of brimstone, herbs, burnt feathers, and other ingredients filled the air. After we had been compelled to endure this stifling atmosphere for four or five minutes, the windows and doors were once more opened. A person of a consumptive habit could scarcely have survived this inhuman ordeal.'[49]

Eventually, fumigation in a lazaretto became almost the stuff of legend. The description given by Merideth Johnes in his didactic book of travel and adventure for boys gives the impression that he had suffered fumigation himself at Beirut. He wrote vividly about new arrivals being taken unawares. When they go to bed,

> 'a horrible, suffocating smoke, and still viler smell, comes floating up stairs, and speedily diffuses itself so completely throughout their rooms, as to set them coughing like steam-engines . . . and compel them to throw open their windows to prevent being stifled. The authorities are fumigating the suspected company with brimstone; to which, in some places, burnt feathers are added, by way of increasing the pungency of the remedy.'[50]

There are, however, enough similarities with passages in Bayard Taylor's *Pictures of Palestine*, published four years earlier, to suggest that Johnes was 'borrowing'.[51]

Travellers in the era of cholera found that fumigation was adopted in desperation, despite a general consensus among doctors that the disease was not contagious in the same way as plague. Captain Frankland, detained at Carlscrona in the Baltic in 1831, learnt that the ship's surgeon was 'to smoke us *daily for thirty days*! We shall be like good hams', he joked, 'before our probation is finished'.[52] Luckily that rumour proved false, but between France and Italy the smoking was real, and travellers were shocked by the unexpected brutality. Arriving at Villa Franca in 1832, Nathaniel Willis was locked for an hour with others in a little round tower in the harbour. The reason for the

> 'delay was presently explained by clouds of smoke issuing from the interior. The tower filled, and a more nauseating odour I never inhaled. We were near suffocating with the intolerable smell and the quantity of smoke deemed necessary . . . against contagion.'[53]

But the master of invective against cholera fumigation was Mark Twain. As late as 1867, in a letter home to his editor written during a European tour, he complained,

> 'We have been fumigated – not once only, but several times – at the Lake of Como, at Lecco, and almost infernally at Venice. We have been fumigated until we smell of all the vile stenches that can be compounded or imagined. Each and every passenger has acquired a distinct and individual odor, and made it his own, and you can recognize any one of them by it in the dark as far as you can smell him.'[54]

He also wrote in his journal, after describing a particularly nasty and unexpected fumigation at Bellaggio, that it was like 'the Black Hole of Calcutta on a small scale'. He was outraged but determined to follow his Christian values, so 'I shall still try to pray for these fumigating, maccaroni-stuffing [*sic*] organ grinders'.[55]

In those ports which practised the *spoglio*, the fumigation of minor personal effects took place while travellers were undressing. Their money and jewellery were immersed in water or in something more sinister. Captain Jesse, at Odessa, 'having delivered over my watch, money, pencil-case, and every other article about me, had the satisfaction of seeing them (with the exception of the former) placed in a solution of chloride of lime'.[56] The choice of chemicals for fumigation was limited: at Rostov-on-Don in 1812, they used 'nitrous muriatic acid, after the method of Guiton de Morvaux';[57] at Odessa they used sulphuric acid as well as chloride of lime;[58] while at Lisbon they produced 'a little crucible in which was a dangerous-looking compound of chloride of lime and various other disinfectants'.[59] Larger baggage was taken away to a fumigation house, where the contents were removed and exposed to a long process of 'depuration'. At Odessa, the cleansing teams

> 'were dressed in suits of coarse leather, and gloves of the same. Their dexterity in opening trunks and finding out secret drawers was quite amusing. The Bramah locks opened as if by magic; and Mr. Chubb would here have lost his premium. Such was the severity of the search . . . that hair in rings, brooches, and lockets, was taken out, and the linings of dressing cases, as well as the carriage cushions ripped open. Every article of metal as well as silk that was submitted to the action of the chloride was injured, and several of my antique lamps in terra cotta were broken.'[60]

As for the clothes removed during the *spoglio*, they were taken at Odessa to one of four large warehouses.

> 'A condemned criminal is employed to hang them up on long spars that run the breadth of the [ware]houses, about fourteen inches apart: he

also turns them several times a week: and at the expiration of forty-two days they are pronounced clean, provided the said criminal remains free from infection.'[61]

Similar treatment, generally for shorter periods, took place at other quarantine stations. At Syra, 'dishes with pots of burning sulphur were placed in each room, and the doors kept closed for half-an-hour'.[62] The process was always thorough, often rough, and locksmiths were consistently humbled as they had been at Odessa. On Malta, Samuel Bevan delivered the keys of his portmanteau to a guardian who 'unceremoniously' tipped out the contents, hanging the clothes on racks.

> 'Nothing escaped his vigilance. Dressing-case and drawing-box were fished out and opened, and the secret recesses of my writing-desk, which it almost puzzled *me* to arrive at, flew apart as if by magic, at the 'open-sesame' of my unnatural guardian, who finished up taking the tops off my pill-boxes, and the stoppers out of my medicine-bottles.'[63]

Another unhappy detainee at Malta was the missionary Maxwell Macbrair. All the bottles had to be unpacked from his medicine chest, their paper wrappers were burnt and the bottles were arranged for airing. Macbrair saw 'such little packages as a few pencils or wafers, or sticks of sealing-wax . . . or a few old letters or tracts tied up together' being 'pulled to pieces' and blamed it all on 'popish Malta'.[64] The American clergyman Justin Perkins had a nasty experience when entering Georgia from Persia in 1834.

> 'My boxes, on which I had bestowed almost endless toil, – having constructed them with my own hands at Constantinople . . . were every one rudely split open and broken to pieces even, and their contents strown [*sic*] over the smoke-house; and thus they were made to lie during the whole period of our quarantine.'[65]

Although watches were spared purification by chemicals, they did not always escape immersion in water. Adolphus Slade would

> 'have preferred having my watch smoked, but the regulations were precise; hydrophobia was inadmissible. It was a Breguet, and passed uninjured through the ordeal. But [his companion] the doctor's timepiece did not perform its functions with regularity after the immersion.'[66]

The scientist Dr Friedrich Parrot hoped that his sensitive instruments would be similarly spared a chemical cleansing when he reached a quarantine station in the Caucasus mountains. But the local physician was unsympathetic. As whole villages were burned when necessary on account of the plague, why should his instruments be spared? Parrot had to work hard for the reasons, arguing first that his observations and recordings would count for nothing if further tests could not be made on his return; secondly, that the instruments were metal which was not a conductor of contagion; and thirdly, that Parrot himself was a physician and had made it his 'sacred duty' to avoid any contact with the plague. He won a partial victory, in that his instruments could be washed with vinegar rather than exposed to the vapour of chlorine.[67]

In the compulsory opening of baggage and effects, there was of course a risk that particularly personal or sensitive items might come to light to the embarrassment or even danger of the owner. Albert Hervey on Malta observed, 'There was one lady amongst our party, who almost fainted, when she heard her boxes were to be turned inside out'.[68] Hervey was intrigued that another passenger 'had a *mummy* from Egypt, nicely packed and soldered in tin, and nailed up in a strong deal case'. The guardians insisted on opening and airing the mummy, 'to prevent contagion, forsooth!' as Hervey aptly exclaimed.[69] Also on Malta, Samuel Bevan was not amused that his effects and those of his fortuitous messmates were littered for airing around their rooms:

> 'each individual's private collection giving a sufficiently good clue to his tastes and character. There were enough of cherry-sticks and chibouques to have stocked a cigar-divan, whilst we might easily have managed a bal-costumé with the variety of Oriental dresses which were here brought to light.'[70]

For one man, however, Bevan had no sympathy. This individual stood red-faced in front of the 'chippings from the glorious temples of Upper Egypt, which had been cracked off during his antiquarian ramble, to serve as trophies and mementoes when he should regain his own fireside'.[71]

The only instance which has come to light of a downright refusal to hand over an item for cleansing occurred at Orsova in 1836. Miss Pardoe, the narrator, was stoical but vexed at the seizure of her own possessions:

> 'they were peculiarly inquisitive; counting my rings, and recording my bracelets and necklaces. Not a pocket-handkerchief, nor a waist-ribbon escaped; and I was more than once asked if I had really exhibited the whole of my wardrobe. My books and drawings were seized without ceremony, and carried off to be examined by the proper officer.'[72]

Gentlemen of the party were asked to deliver up their guns (not usually a requirement in lazarettos), and then a British colonel was asked to surrender his sword. This was too much. The officer roared with anger 'that he would fell to the earth the first man who dared to meddle with his side-arms'. The guardian insisted, but the soldier stood his ground. The guardian (who was armed with a pistol) then retreated and reported the incident to the governor, who chose to do nothing.[73]

If the guardian at Orsova was taken aback by this arrogance, health officials on Malta nearly 200 years earlier had been shocked for a different reason. The Roman traveller Pietro della Valle arrived at Valletta in 1625. He had some trouble with his own bill of health, which was less precise and lucid than that of the ship which had brought him from Cyprus. Health guardians wanted to know more about '*la balle de fil*' in his possession, but della Valle was cagey about what it contained. Later he was allowed ashore and underwent his quarantine by special favour in grand private lodgings, where he was nevertheless obliged to deliver his effects. In '*une grande gallerie couverte*' attached to the house, his clothes and possessions were spread out for airing. When it came to the mystery bale, there was still the coy reluctance of della Valle to open it, but he told the guardians what was within – the body of his dead wife which he was passionate to return to Italy. Shocked officials explained that unless and until it was aired, there was no question of him being given a clean bill of health for the onward voyage. After appeal to higher authority, della Valle won his battle. It was accepted that opening the bale would harm the corpse, and as long as he would swear as to all the circumstances of the death, and particularly that it was not plague related, he could have his bill of health.[74] The issue for Malta was delicate because, if the existence of this body in quarantine was leaked, Sicily would embargo all trade with Malta and the vital grain ships, which stopped the Maltese from starving, would immediately cease.

Given the progress of medicine in the nineteenth century, it seems odd that in some ports the necessity for fumigation continued. But plague never quite disappeared from the Near East, so health authorities were reluctant to break with tradition, while those affected were increasingly disinclined to put up with it. The result was a mere going through the motions – a token cleansing to assuage the conscience of a board of health and soothe the rebellious humour of those detained. The arrival of the large yacht *Griffin* at Alexandria from Syria in 1881 exemplified the problem. Plague in Baghdad meant three days of quarantine in Egypt, with fumigation on the last.

> 'A boat came alongside with a batch of quarantine officials and their followers. Three large earthenware bowls, having been placed near the companion-ladder, were filled with a stinking concoction of sulphur and water, and were then gravely carried through every part of the ship, from the engine-room to the forecastle, after which the horrid mixture was sprinkled everywhere. Our worthy Scotch captain's face was a picture.'[75]

All the crew and passengers were then assembled on deck and told to march past a bowl of burning sulphur. The ladies simply refused, so the bowls were marched past them. After the third day of quarantine, the yacht was presented with a bill for £15, which the Commodore refused to pay for an 'abominable farce'. But in the end he had to, or the yacht would have been impounded.[76]

Once through the fumigation process, new arrivals were allotted a room or rooms in the accommodation block. The average inland lazaretto, as at Orsova, was 'a sort of box within a box' with a square garden in the middle and a promenade within the outer wall.[77] At seaports, topography had more influence on the layout, which could be fan-shaped, as at Aegina, but more probably rectangular or square if the site was less constricted. At Malta the demand for rooms was such that the lazaretto proper was supplemented by nearby Fort Manoel. In the most-frequented ports the conditions were not too harsh, but some of the makeshift lazarettos in the Levant and along the Danube left much to be desired. Only at Malta were the rooms so large that scarcely anyone complained of being cooped up, and some people there were even allocated a suite. It was usually necessary to share accommodation, and it was in the interest of lone travellers to invite acquaintances made during the voyage to join them for the detention. This often resulted in a multinational mix. The Frenchman Raoul de Malherbe found himself among entirely Englishmen on his return voyage from Egypt and had no difficulty associating with them in the lazaretto at Malta.[78] Also at Malta, the English scholar John Gadsby joined up with Americans, having slept in the same cabin as five of them on the ship and having 'no desire to have more agreeable companions than four of them were', which raises an intriguing question about the fifth.[79] At Odessa, Adolphus Slade teamed up with a German doctor, and they altruistically invited a German artisan and a Turkish Jew to join them because the latter two could not afford the expenses.[80]

At other times, company was enforced. Sir Moses Montefiore recorded a night at Syra lazaretto sleeping nine to a room, but those were exceptional circumstances and the following day his small party was given 'the apartments set aside for noblemen'.[81] Enforced sharing was obviously risky. As Captain Best observed, 'One disagreeable person will render a quarantine life horrible'.[82] But most people made an effort to get along. The Abbé de Binos arrived at Leghorn in 1779 and found himself quartered with self-styled royalty from Bactria, an Anglo-American sea captain and a German officer who had recently returned from a royal mission to Turkey.[83] They got on famously, but others were less lucky. Peter Holthaus, a German tailor, was shut up in the Malta lazaretto with a 78-year-old Italian, who whined that he needed to be fed by his roommate and shouted with anger if the food did not suit.[84] At Odessa, Charles Terry was billeted with a Russian officer's servant who got up at dawn,

> 'took a little mirror, and put himself in a corner of my room where I could see him, while he thought I was asleep. He was earnestly candle-tallowing his hair . . . rubbing his Russian pomatum well into his scanty short-cropped bristles. He was a considerable time getting . . . to show

> off to the greatest advantage his singularly piggish face. I could scarcely help laughing outright.'[85]

But these anecdotes are as nothing when compared with the reminiscences of Pierre de Saumery at Leghorn in 1724, for whom the captive hordes inspired visions of Noah's Ark: '*jamais l'arche de Noé n'a renfermé des animaux si variés, ni si differens*', with resulting chaos, quarrels and even murder among those whom the authorities had lumped together.[86]

Many westerners expressed their xenophobia at being forced to mingle with certain races or indeed at the threat of it. The main complaint was alleged uncleanliness. At Calorash on the Danube, the Revd Nathanael Burton was placed in a room with a family of Jews. He held both the family and their race in some respect, so 'overlooked the multifarious nastiness with which they abounded'.[87] Captain Jesse found himself at Odessa among

> 'Russians, Jews, Tartars, Greeks, Sclavonians, and Levanters of all descriptions, evidently living in a deplorable state of ignorance as to the value of soap and water; and the effluvia arising from the close contact of so many dirty people in a badly ventilated room, was enough to produce the very disease which the authorities were taking such pains to prevent us from introducing.'[88]

The American William Cullen Bryant was equally dismissive of pilgrims and dervishes at Gaza 'sleeping in the sun, and picking the vermin – the lice, if you must have the word – from the inside of their garments'.[89] But the most consistent critics were the British military from India, such as Albert Hervey, who refused to leave the steamer at Malta in 1843 'to be packed up in a dirty Lazaretto amongst dirty Turks, Arabs and Armenians'.[90]

Another cause of complaint was lack of furnishings, for instance, at the Old Lazaretto in Venice in 1691: 'When a Man comes to lodge in one of these Rooms, he finds nothing but Four bare Walls, and must therefore buy an entire Set of necessary Furniture'.[91] It was not unusual, even 150 years later, to find bare rooms in some of the remoter lazarettos, but furniture could always be hired from a local inn. In the busier centres the traveller could expect at least a bedstead, table and chair, but they might well be filthy and rickety. It was usually recommended to contact a local hotelier for whatever extra furniture the traveller felt necessary or could afford. At the well-organized lazaretto in Malta, the Garcin Brothers of Valletta produced a published list of furniture for hire at eight pence per day for nine items, including an iron bedstead with mosquito curtain, linen and a dressing table with mirror. Items of relative luxury were much more expensive: a sofa, for instance, cost five shillings for the duration of the quarantine.[92]

At Orsova, Hans Christian Andersen noticed that before each quarantine compartment there was a little slate which noted in chalk 'the day and hour that the stranger was placed there, the day and hour they were to go out, and how many there were in'.[93] There was nothing private about that, and it gave the impression of being penned in a labelled cage, as in a zoo. In fact, the word zoo sprang instantly to mind in other lazarettos, both from the labelling and the succession of little enclosures. At Odessa, Charles Terry confessed,

> 'It is pleasant to get out of our cage, which in every respect resembles a menagerie. There are twenty compartments in the range of the quarantine houses on our side, all with double high wooden gratings, and ticketed, as . . . is done in England to denote a hyena from Egypt, a lion from Barbary, or a bear from Russia.'[94]

Shirley Brooks went along with that:

> 'the arrangement is that of some of the dens in the Zoological Gardens, an effect increased by a species of narrow piazza in front of the compartments, which slightly screens a person, standing close to the bars, from the weather.'[95]

And Charles Henry Scott, also in Odessa, was even more specific: 'a series of dens, precisely like those occupied by the wild beasts of the Zoological Gardens, Regent's Park, and separated from the public by three partitions of iron grating'.[96]

The same feeling of being an exhibit bothered Francis Hervé at Semlin. The lazaretto 'struck me as looking like a menagerie, only instead of birds and beasts peeping through the cages, they were men and women'.[97] Again at Semlin, the Revd George Gleig echoed even more precisely the description of Odessa by mentioning, 'cells . . . resembling the cages of wild beasts in the Zoological gardens'.[98] Julia Pardoe at the Orsova lazaretto found 'the incarcerated individuals amusing themselves by rocking to and fro behind the bars of their prison-gates, and roaring like wild beasts in a menagerie'.[99] In summary, there could be something dehumanizing about the quarantine experience if the public was allowed close enough to see the detainees.

Each traveller when alone, or each group in the case of a shared room, was continually monitored by a *guardiano*, or health guardian, whose job was to prevent any unauthorized or compromising behaviour. This person might share the cell with the detainee, sometimes sleeping on the table, or he might camp immediately outside the door. In the case of a group, there could be more than one guardian, and the relationship with the detainees was frequently awkward to say the least. The guardians most favoured by inmates were old soldiers and sailors (some of them still bearing wounds) because they had a broad view of life and an innate respect for rank. Captain Rochfort Scott was particularly amused by his guardian in the lazaretto at Candia in Crete. Although a Sicilian by birth, the man had served in gunboats of the Royal Navy and 'picked up many choice expressions'. He had also gained a liking for rum, and after every affectionate discourse on the British, he would end with a eulogy on '*quel buon grog*'.[100]

Occasionally, guardians acted like a servant or batman, tidying the room, laying the table and brushing clothes. But more often than not he 'was a stupid old fellow', indolent and rather petulant, with annoying habits like smoking and spitting.[101] The worst guardians could make quarantine a misery. Jean Dumont lamented his experience at Venice in 1691, where 'we have the Misfortune to be plagu'd with one who mortifies us extremely'.[102] At Leghorn, in 1725, guardians were slated as '*de veritables monstres*'.[103] At Civitavecchia, in 1806, two sailors were put on board ship as guardians, there being no lazaretto on shore. Edward Dodwell was 'disgusted with the abandoned, revolting, and blasphemous behaviour of these miscreants, who were far less civilized, and much more wicked than our late companions the thieves of Ithaca'.[104] It was almost as bad to be landed with a guardian who was simply quirky. At Semlin on the Danube, Francis Hervé was startled to see his guardian enter one day in fancy dress, but as the man's wife did their washing for a fee – although not the ironing – he was reluctant to make a scene.[105] On the Persian-Russian border, General Alexander Macintosh was kept awake all night by his guardian who was 'talking to himself and singing in the low tremulous style of the country, and occasionally uttering groans, yawns, and exclamations, and even laughing by turns, as different humours seized him'.[106]

One reason for friction with guardians, and indeed with higher ranks in certain lazarettos, was the language barrier. This was not a problem in the main western ports where officials often spoke several languages, as indeed did the travellers. A working knowledge of French in western Europe, Italian in the Levant and German in the Balkans and Caucasus prevented many misunderstandings, and of course English was spoken predominantly in the lazarettos on Malta and the Ionian Islands. At Semlin lazaretto, an official interpreter was on the payroll, which was most unusual.[107] At Odessa, where Italian was the lingua franca, the quarantine officer seemed able to talk to every nationality in their own language.[108] But guardians often spoke only their native tongue, and in some places the authorities were indifferent to the problems which inevitably arose. At Constantinople, as late as 1842, no language was spoken or understood by the guardians except Turkish, which most travellers found impenetrable.[109]

One of the worst experiences in communication was suffered by the Revd Charles Elliott, vicar of Godalming, at the crossing of the River Pruth from Moldavia into Russian-held Bessarabia. Elliott was no mean linguist, but the episode degenerated into farce when he was asked to take an oath written in Russian, which he did not understand. A Jew offered to translate it into English, but the Russians were against this, alleging that a Jew could not mention Christ without committing blasphemy. 'The absurdity of this conversation was the more glaring', wrote Elliott, 'as a Jew was at the time actually naming the name of Christ in his office of interpreter between us'.[110]

Elliott was unlucky, as there were people in the nearby town who might well have assisted, but the Russians had no wish to make it easy. As the nineteenth century progressed, British tourists lost the facility of their forbears to master French and Italian, the basic languages of travel. This put them at a serious disadvantage in the Near East, where they 'were subjected to every imaginable evil' by their guides and guardians.[111]

The innkeeper or hotelier who supplied the furniture could usually be called upon to provide the food, but the larger lazarettos employed a restaurateur, also known as a *spenditore*. At Orsova, the restaurant attached to the lazaretto provided bedding as well as food. The status of a restaurateur was not always apparent. He could have won a contract from the management of the lazaretto, or he could be a government appointee. Few of them were as bizarre as the monopolist at Aintab in southern Turkey, who had

> 'grown fat in his office, and, unlike his stores, was fresh and full weight. He could neither write nor read, so kept the accounts of his customers on a large sheet of paper, and these were distinguished by rude representations of some peculiarity of their persons. . . . Horizontal lines indicated the amount of piastres the customer had paid on account, and perpendicular the number of paras.'[112]

In contrast to this was the slick *trattoria* instituted within the Malta lazaretto in 1838. The idea was not unique, as Marseilles and Leghorn had developed similar institutions, but at Malta there was a range of printed menus arranged by price and the well-off could even hire their own cook.

As prices in the Maltese *trattoria* were advertised in sterling, the British traveller knew what was value for money. Few would have jibbed at a breakfast of tea, coffee, milk, bread, butter and hot or cold meat for one shilling and eight pence, or a dinner of soup, fish or meat, vegetables, a dessert, cheese, fruit, bread and a bottle of Sicilian wine for four shillings. A detainee on a budget could have a lesser dinner for two shillings and sixpence. The wine list carried 27 options ranging from champagne at five shillings and four pence a bottle, via claret, rum and ale, to the cheapest item – a bottle of Portuguese Faro wine for one shilling.[113] This *trattoria*, championed by both the Maltese superintendent of quarantine and the British island governor, would have opened sooner if there had not been a problem with relocating the coal store for steamers, which threatened all areas of the lazaretto with a penetrating and polluting dust.[114]

Across quarantine ports as a whole, differences in the quality and diversity of provisions were profound, but it was by no means an East-West split. Customer satisfaction at Malta and Trieste was equalled by matchless fruit and vegetables at Gaza, while at Beirut the soup was 'liquified bliss', and a dish of larks left its American consumer asking divine forgiveness for regretting 'that more songs had not been silenced' in the preparation.[115] At Jerusalem, in 1843, Dawson Borrer marvelled at the 'most dainty-looking dish of fricasée' placed before him, spoilt only by the lump of old cloth which suddenly appeared on the end of his fork.[116] At Sevastopol, beef was just 'a penny a pound, and the best we ever tasted out of England', confessed Adolphus Slade.[117] But in many of the smaller lazarettos, the food might be simply disgusting, depending on the season, the availability of produce, the time of the day and the distance a meal had to travel. The inn could be a mile away, as at Semlin, so the dinner was 'greasy and cold' on arrival.[118] At Orsova, Hans Christian Andersen endured sour cabbage, fat pork and Danube water, but at least it was on the premises.[119]

The priority for newcomers was to understand the limits of their freedom, which meant coming to terms with the rules of contagion. Quarantine worked on the principle that certain items were intrinsically liable to spread disease while certain others were not. Curiously, Venice, which had been so strict in early years, became uniquely tolerant. In the seventeenth century, an inmate in the new lazaretto could exchange bread, wine, tobacco, wood and money with persons in pratique 'and generally every thing that does not consist of Threads'.[120] That laxity would have appalled officials at other ports, but at least there was consensus about fibres. All items of clothing and soft furnishing were automatically suspect, and the definition of threads included paper. By the mid-nineteenth century, despite advances in science, anomalies remained. Money, unless dipped in water or vinegar, could not be accepted from anyone even remotely suspected of plague. Yet, at any date it was possible to write an order for supplies on slate, which could travel to and from a local inn without causing fear as the surface was deemed too hard for 'particles' of plague to cling to it.[121]

Another job of the guardian was to ensure that his charge did not at any time touch anyone in pratique or any person within the lazaretto who had arrived at a later date. For a breach of the former rule, a compromised person from outside would have been held two weeks in quarantine, and in the second instance the period of detention of the person touching would have been lengthened to include that of the touched. Yet there were circumstances, for instance on the excursions from Semlin to Belgrade or in a perambulation of the grounds of a lazaretto (where such grounds existed), when other people were very much in range. Newcomers to quarantine, despite warnings in guidebooks, were sometimes so amazed at the antics of those who sought to avoid them that they misconstrued the motive. Francis Hervé at Semlin, seeing people backing away as he approached, 'thought what a very polite people they must be, or how very imposing my appearance, to command so much obsequiousness'.[122] Those who understood the pantomime best had usually spent some time in Egypt, where plague was endemic. Joseph Sherer summed up the scene:

> 'To those who have never been in a plague-infected city, and have never seen a case of plague . . . it is at first highly comic to see all the little precautions adopted; and you cannot meet without a smile those Franks,

> whose more humble rank, or the nature of their business, compels to stir about, armed with a thick stick to prevent a dog touching them, and making wide circuits *to windward*, round every man, camel, and jackass, which they meet.'[123]

As there was no exemption from the rules for lazaretto staff, guardians were as much in quarantine as their charges whom they never touched. At Rothenturn, the Revd Robert Walsh walked about with a guardian who was dressed like an undertaker and carried a long pole to ward off the detainees. 'Whenever we accidentally approached, he dilated his staring eyes, waved his staff between us, and uttered, in German, a long and loud expostulation'. When his cloak brushed against Walsh in a gust of wind, he held 'the guilty flap at the end of his staff . . . [and] hastened down and purified it in the river'.[124]

The captain of the lazaretto at Malta was allegedly detained in his own institution, having been accidentally grazed by the parasol of a lady inmate.[125] Even indirect contact was deemed highly dangerous. Samuel Bevan, also at Malta, wrote that he

> 'was severely reprimanded for having scattered some torn fragments of letters from my window, as, had the breeze been sufficiently strong to carry any portion over the water . . . I should innocently have placed the whole island in quarantine.'[126]

In the same lazaretto, the guardians noticed that a slipper fell from a balcony and hit the restaurateur, whom

> 'they fell upon . . . like the angels of punishment. The poor man ran away to his boat, where he touched the other two that were with him. . . . All three were brought up and obliged to perform the quarantine.'[127]

Hans Christian Andersen, in the Orsova lazaretto, recalled,

> 'We had to look about us, and see that the wind did not bring a little feather over the wall, that might fall on our shoulders; – see that we did not tread on a thread that any one had lost; – for in that case, the quarantine was lengthened.'[128]

On the island of Zante, trees were felled in case birds made nests in them with unpurified cotton taken from the lazaretto.[129]

The anecdote of the good-natured butcher shows how the ordinary traveller might be the ultimate victim of this over-caution. In 1854, this man was aboard a steamer at Malta heading east, watching six horses being lowered into a lighter for ferrying ashore. The animals had suffered on the voyage, inducing the butcher to jump down to cover them with horse cloths. But the lighter was technically in quarantine, so that if the butcher returned to the steamer he would compromise the ship, meriting ten days' quarantine for everyone at Alexandria. He was horrified 'and, with a very long face . . . entered the health-boat, and was at once rowed off to the Lazaretto, where, as long as daylight remained, he was seen looking wistfully towards the ship'.[130] Incidentally, the same steamer was not allowed to draw water on board at Malta, as the hosepipe would have established 'a connection' between ship and shore.[131]

Notes

See general note as to references stated at the end of Chapter 1.

1 *Hansard's Parliamentary Debates*, lxxvi (London, 1844), 1305.
2 Laurent (1821, 84).
3 Beauvau, de (1619, 172).
4 Valle (1745, viii, 173).
5 Saumery (1732–5, 84–5).
6 Woods (1828, ii, 308).
7 Montefiore (1836, 262–3).
8 Ibid., 272.
9 Damer (1841, ii, 254–5).
10 Scott (1900, v, 370). The reference to 'Spanish' is puzzling, and it is possible Scott was confined in the best rooms in Fort Manoel.
11 Najaf (1839, i, 213).
12 Vane (1842, ii, 35); cf. Vane (1844, 166–7); she called the four rooms 'miserable'.
13 Vane (1844, 194).
14 Sutherland (1790, 260–1).
15 Woburn Abbey Collection, 6th Duke, MS. Diary 3/21/3.
16 Scott (1853, 758).
17 *British Parliamentary Papers* (1843, liv, 36–7).
18 Howel (1788, 155).
19 Grellet (1860, ii, 44).
20 Cambridge University Library, MSS Dept., Add. MS. 7633/1/86.
21 Caroline (1821, 698).
22 Biddle (1993, 195).
23 Marmont (1837, iii, 124–6).
24 Keppel (1827, ii, 257).
25 Burgess (1835, ii, 288).
26 Ibid.
27 Dreux (1925, 182).
28 Jesse (1841, i, 56).
29 Ibid., i, 57.
30 Slade (1840, 310).
31 Ibid.
32 Ibid., 310–11.
33 Ibid., 311.
34 Terry (1848, 246–7).
35 Burton (1838, 270).
36 Slade (1840, 312).
37 Stephens (1839, i, 262–3).
38 Terry (1848, 247).

39 Macgill (1808, ii, 185).
40 Macbrair (1839, 118).
41 Wilkinson (1843, i, 54); cf. Slatter (1984, 79).
42 Galton (1908, 55).
43 Stephens (1839, i, 261).
44 Laurent (1821, 254).
45 Saumery (1732–5, iv, 135–9).
46 Ibid., iv, 149.
47 Plaisted (1757, 150).
48 Grellet (1860, i, 114).
49 Pfeiffer (1852, 218).
50 Johnes (1859, 137–8).
51 cf. Taylor (1855, 25).
52 Frankland (1832, ii, 457).
53 Willis (1850, 8–9).
54 Twain (1958, 75).
55 Twain (1875, 199–200).
56 Jesse (1841, i, 56).
57 Freygang (1823, 255).
58 Stephens (1839, i, 263).
59 Browne (1867, 309).
60 Jesse (1841, i, 60–1).
61 Pinkerton (1833, 132).
62 Montefiore (1890, i, 263).
63 Bevan (1849, 162).
64 Macbrair (1839, 191–2).
65 Perkins (1843, 124).
66 Slade (1840, 308).
67 Parrot (1845, 261–2).
68 Hervey (1846, ii, 72).
69 Ibid., 73–4.
70 Bevan (1849, 162).
71 Ibid., 162–3.
72 Pardoe (1854, 333).
73 Ibid.
74 Valle (1745, viii, 167–75).
75 Maxwell (1882, 83–5).
76 Ibid.
77 Andersen (1846, iii, 169).
78 Malherbe (1846, ii, 386–90).
79 Gadsby (1880, 540).
80 Slade (1840, 312).
81 Montefiore (1890, i, 263).
82 Best (1842, 320).
83 Binos (1798, ii, 355).
84 Holthaus (1844, 262–3).
85 Terry (1848, 253–4).
86 Saumery (1732–5, iv, 145).
87 Burton (1838, 269).
88 Jesse (1841, i, 54).
89 Bryant (1869, 164).
90 Hervey (1846, ii, 67).
91 Dumont (1705, 350).

92 Wilkinson (1847, xxii–xxiii).
93 Andersen (1846, iii, 172).
94 Terry (1848, 254).
95 Brooks (1854, 30).
96 Scott (1854, 339).
97 Hervé (1837, ii, 320).
98 Gleig (1839, iii, 277).
99 Pardoe (1854, 333).
100 Scott (1837, ii, 252–3).
101 Woods (1828, ii, 307).
102 Dumont (1705, 350).
103 Saumery (1732–5, iv, 141).
104 Dodwell (1819, ii, 467).
105 Hervé (1837, ii, 332).
106 Macintosh (1854, ii, 72).
107 Hervé (1837, ii, 327): 'He was a fine gentlemanly fellow, a Hungarian by birth, and held his appointment under the Austrian government'.
108 Stephens (1839, i, 261).
109 Fisk (1844, 417).
110 Elliott (1838, i, 223).
111 Neale (1852, i, 19).
112 Walpole (1851, i, 254–5).
113 National Archives of Malta, C1, pp. 314–16.
114 Ibid., pp. 260–63; Booker (2007, 523–4).
115 Taylor (1855, 21).
116 Borrer (1845, 398).
117 Slade (1854, 259).
118 Keppel (1831, i, 461).
119 Andersen (1846, iii, 169).
120 Dumont (1705, 350).
121 For example, see Waring (1843, 58) and Baxter (1850, 271).
122 Hervé (1837, ii, 330).
123 Sherer (1825, 197–8).
124 Walsh (1829, 309–10).
125 Damer (1841, ii, 255).
126 Bevan (1849, 164).
127 Najaf (1839, i, 216–17).
128 Andersen (1846, iii, 173).
129 Minet (1958, 267).
130 Beaumont (1856, i, 46).
131 Ibid., 41.

4 Passing the time

During a long quarantine, despite efforts to make one day different from another, the traveller inevitably fell into a routine. Boredom soon brought into focus the proclivities of gender and nationality.

One French detainee summed up an average day in the Malta lazaretto: the women were sentimental and read novels; the Italians boasted of their conquests; the Germans spent much of the day and some of the night smoking; the English drank champagne; and the French managed to sing and talk politics at the same time.[1] But even this does not quite capture the variety and ingenuity of keeping busy. Apart from letter writing, the most obvious time-filler was the upkeep of a diary or journal, an occupation which the guidebooks recommended. In fact, confinement was conducive to any kind of writing, and Benjamin Disraeli, while in quarantine at Malta, is believed to have written much of *Contarini Fleming* and *Alroy*.[2] Drawing, sketching and painting were equally popular, and the picturesque situation of many lazarettos gave inspiration for new subjects, as well as allowing time for existing works to be retouched. Charles Monk, quarantined in Palestine, 'had occasion twenty times a day to regret my inability to carry Hebron, its picturesque scenes and views, away with me in a sketch-book. The pencil of a sister would have been invaluable'.[3]

Another cerebral pastime was reading. The Revd Thomas Smart Hughes, quarantined at Barletta, 'read through the entire works of Horace in his native province', while the theologian Robert Pinkerton finished a two-volume German treatise on Luther and the Reformation among the works he devoured at Odessa.[4] As Pinkerton was then in his fourth 'quarantine imprisonment', he had no doubt exhausted all other pastimes. John Carne, on Zante, read Byron in intervals between drinking the local wine.[5] Many travellers brought books along with them or were supplied with well-worn editions by local contacts. In the larger lazarettos, especially Malta, reading material was readily available. Mrs Montefiore recorded her thanks to 'Lady Stoddart, who brought a box of books for our amusement'.[6] Mrs Lucinda Griffith was delighted to 'have a good supply of books from the garrison library at Valetta, to which we subscribe, whose liberal arrangements afforded us an easy access to all the newest publications'.[7] At the same

DOI: 10.4324/9781003195733-5

lazaretto, John Kinnear noted that 'a circulating-library offers its bill of fare as soon as your arrival is known', possibly 'Muir's Library' mentioned by Samuel Bevan.[8] Again on Malta, the French consul could supply even the newest French books to his fellow citizens.[9] One of the inconsistencies of quarantine was that the handling of books was not treated with the same precautionary fumigation as the transfer of letters. Only at the Rothenturn lazaretto, in the 1820s, was there any mention of formality. There, some novels of Sir Walter Scott translated into French were lent to the Revd Robert Walsh by another inmate: 'a man with a wooden tray on a pole thrust them in at the window'.[10]

Most detainees wanted newspapers to catch up with social and political change. When Edward Ives arrived at Leghorn in 1758, the British consul wrote, 'I am sorry I cannot send you any *English* papers; the officers of the navy have carried them all away, but the bearer brings you some *French Leyden* gazettes'.[11] The most sought-after newspaper was the reputable Galignani's *Messenger*, an English-language daily published in Paris. William Drew Stent, incarcerated in a lazaretto close to Constantinople in 1842, welcomed 'a pile' of them from a former travelling companion, while a few years later Robert Heywood was promised 'Galignani and milk, food for mind and body' from the English consulate in the Dardanelles.[12] At Piraeus, the Earl of Carlisle welcomed 'a batch of Galignanis' to enliven his quarantine before visiting Athens.[13] The usefulness of the paper can be judged by the remarks of Lady Grosvenor, who arrived at Malta in 1841. In the quarantine harbour, her party was greeted by Sir Hector Greig, Chief Secretary to the Governor and a former head of the quarantine service. Greig

> 'gave us the last series of Galignani, arrived by the "Prometheus" steamer this morning from Marseilles, with the account of the new ministerial arrangements consequent upon the resignation of Lord Melbourne's government and the assumption of office by Sir Robert Peel.'[14]

In 1827, Judith Montefiore, while also at Malta, learnt from a Galignani of the marriage of her brother Isaac to Sarah Samuel.[15] And it was not only Galignanis which were available. At Odessa, in 1836, Edmund Spencer thanked 'kind friends, who supplied me with every thing I could desire, including what was indeed most welcome, – not only the latest English periodical publications, but some of the latest daily papers'.[16] At Smyrna, the American priest Stephen Olin was lucky enough to receive newspapers from his homeland from missionaries who visited him in the lazaretto.[17]

Unlike books, newspapers merited a fear of contagion similar to letters, but it is not evident from the examples just quoted that precautions were always taken. When Colonel Fitzclarence arrived at Malta in 1818, he received 'a number of French and English newspapers' from the authorities but was warned not to let a loose sheet blow away as it would inflict quarantine on anyone it touched.[18] John Kinnear was made all too aware of the danger from newspapers in 1839, when he suffered from a strict interpretation of the rules which he could hardly have foreseen. The captain of the ship in which he had arrived at Malta

> 'called for me yesterday and brought some English newspapers, which he tossed across the barrier, and I very thoughtlessly picked up and put in my pocket; and my quarantine has, in consequence, been extended two days, the ship having two days longer than the passengers.'[19]

Some quarantine inmates used their time imaginatively. John Henry Newman practised the violin, wrote verse and studied Italian.[20] In later years, Stendhal advocated learning a new language in quarantine and recommended the works of Hume for the study of English and those of Pignotti for Italian.[21] He advised learning by heart one page during the day and another at night, which would impart enough wisdom after 20 days to allow a novel to be read with ease. Violins and pianos could be hired at Malta, and at Odessa 'a couple of musical boxes' were obtained from the town along with books and playing cards.[22] On the subject of cards, gambling was rife in the Malta lazaretto, although relatively few Britons indulged in the practice. An English visitor noted: 'The gaming-table was established, as usual, by the foreigners; and heavy were the fluctuations of fortune, if we might judge from the changeful demeanour of those who frequented it'.[23] Heavy they certainly were. Jean Giraudeau reckoned that if some games had gone on any longer, several of his party would have been rendered destitute. When not busy with playing cards, they enjoyed a more innovative form of gambling. As soon as a fly was detected in the room, each person put a sugar cube on the table, and wagers were taken as to whose cube the fly would settle on first. This was known as '*la course aux mouches*', and the betting was serious.[24]

The opportunity for sport, and indeed for exercise of any kind, depended entirely on the location. There was no scope at all at Leghorn or Ancona, and even at Marseilles where quarantine was particularly long, nothing was permitted beyond a wander within the confines of the lazaretto. Such internal inspection could take some time – up to three hours in the case of Malta – but was hardly exercise. One of the few points, however, to compensate for bad conditions in the remoter lazarettos was the possibility of a hike in the countryside. General Macintosh was allowed to leave the quarantine camp on the River Aras, between Persia and Russia, to visit the historic, ruined city of Julfa (or Djulfa), which lay a short journey upstream.[25] At Rothenturn, the Revd Robert Walsh wandered through the mountains of Transylvania with his guardian a few paces behind:

> 'we fell into a broad path, which passed over the highest ridge like a good road. . . . On each side were steep wooded precipices; and below,

an infinite variety of deep glens with small rivers running through them, dividing the ridges of hill into the most tortuous and fantastic shapes.'[26]

With excursions like that, some of the deprivations of quarantine could appear inconsequential.

Another mountain wanderer was Robert Heywood, who was in the amazingly relaxed lazaretto of Kavak on the Asiatic shore of the Bosphorus, with a view to the Black Sea. Day after day he rose early in the morning for his three-hour ramble apparently without a guardian, reaching an old castle 'through shady walks scented by old fallen leaves of the bay tree', while nibbling at filberts, teasing tortoises and then settling down in a ruined tower or a crumbling wall for a view of the gulls and porpoises.[27] At least it made up for the rats in the lazaretto itself. At Odessa it was also possible to walk in the countryside every day, albeit under guard, but few inmates would have wished to do that in the south Russian winter. One rare instance of similar freedom is recorded at Otranto, where John Bramsen 'obtained permission to walk out in the fields to respire the fresh air, but always under condition of being followed by our persecuting attendant'.[28]

An unusual form of exercise was boating. There was an instance at Odessa in 1835 of 'leave to row about the harbour in a boat',[29] but the privilege was rare and unheard of in the main western lazarettos with the exception of Malta. The history of boat trips from the Malta lazaretto is not straightforward. The practice of what Judith Montefiore called 'boat-airing'[30] appears to have begun in the 1820s and was a popular pastime in the following decade. John Auldjo was a typical enthusiast: 'we were allowed to row about the harbour, and amuse ourselves in any other way we liked, from daybreak until night . . . sometimes we took a row out to sea'.[31] The water posed no discernible risk to public health, but approaching too close to land was considered dangerous. The Frenchman Marchebeus and his several acquaintances from the same steamer hired ten boats, each with a yellow flag, and were advised that if they went beyond certain limits the guards of the lazaretto would open fire.[32]

This was also the warning to George Waring, a naturalist, who nevertheless persuaded his guardian to let him land in isolated places. One pebbly foreshore, nestling between projecting angles of the Valletta fortifications, he nicknamed Chiton Beach from the number of such shells which abounded there.[33] But he was not always allowed to land at the same spot, nor was he permitted to lean out of the boat to pick a plant or even to fish. As no reason was forthcoming for the fishing ban, Waring concluded sarcastically 'that a fish, having taken a bait which had been touched by a person in quarantine, might escape, and communicate an infectious disease to all the other fish in the harbour'.[34] John Kinnear was allowed to fish from the lazaretto as long as it was before six o'clock in the morning – an equally baffling regulation which amounted in his view 'to a prohibition'.[35]

Despite restrictions within the quarantine basin, Auldjo was not the only man to row out of its mouth. Count Joseph D'Estourmel was allowed, as a special favour, to row around to the Grand Harbour in Valletta.[36] But at some point in the next year or so, an unidentified Englishman took advantage of this relative freedom to communicate unlawfully with some ships, and the privilege of boating was instantly withdrawn. It was not, however, an absolute ban. When ambassador Rashid Pasha passed though the Malta lazaretto in 1838, his sons were allowed the use of a rowing boat. Unfortunately for the Maltese authorities, the British anti-contagionist Arthur Holroyd was in the lazaretto at the same time and petitioned for a similar privilege. Governor Bouverie refused, stating that that the concession to the boys was on the condition that no one else claimed it as a precedent for themselves, in which case the boat would be withdrawn from the children. Holroyd replied that he had no wish to deprive them of their fun, but the new rule rested on the fear of contagion and so waiving it under any circumstance was illogical.[37] This became material for anti-contagionist propaganda, as four years later John Bowring raised the incident in the House of Commons.[38]

After Holroyd's intervention, the privilege of boating returned, but only slowly. In 1840, T.H. Usborne wrote that,

> 'Neither at Malta nor Trieste could we prevail on the authorities to grant us a boat to get a little fresh air . . . with the exception, at the former place, of allowing us to be rowed to the quarantine burial-ground, – not the most charming sight in the world for those incarcerated in the Lazarette.'[39]

Lucinda Griffith, a few years later, was even more upset:

> 'I begged to have one of the pretty little awning boats I saw rowing about the harbour, and thought one was secured for me, when, to my dismay, I found the only use we were to be allowed to make of it was, that it should tow us by a long cord in a miserable open boat, as the awning might carry infection.'[40]

Others were more fortunate. In 1845, Walter Watson was allowed to row in the quarantine ground, setting out from his steamer which was anchored there.[41] Two years later, John Gadsby 'sometimes took a boat, and, accompanied by a guardian, rowed about the harbour'.[42] But Cuthbert Young, also in 1847, found life more complicated: 'One day we were rowed round the little bay, having to engage two boats for the purpose, as the rowers were not allowed to sit near us'.[43] This was also the system in the Grand Harbour of Valletta, as Albert Hervey discovered. 'If we wished to take a row in the harbour', wrote Hervey, 'we were all put into one boat, with a guardiana at the bows holding a yellow flag, and towed about by another boat'.[44]

Swimming was another activity permitted at Malta, but rarely elsewhere. John Kinnear found that his bathing, like his fishing, had to be done before six in the morning.[45] George Waring thought swimming 'delightful', although the locals warned him against it as the sea was too cold in December.[46] Jean Giraudeau was sure of the advantages in the height of summer: '*La natation était pour nous un besoin d'hygiène et une partie de plaisir*'.[47] But considering that the quarantine harbour was relatively enclosed and received the effluent of the lazaretto as well as of part of the town, the hygienic side was possibly an illusion. When the weather was hot enough, in any event, the health risk was disregarded. According to Marchebeus, when the temperature on Malta reached 30 degrees Celsius, bathing was the only way to get by.[48] The swimming allowed from the lazaretto of Beirut was no doubt rather cleaner, as the site was swept by the open sea.[49]

More extreme activities were not impossible, but the traveller needed to be in a remote lazaretto with a tolerant regime. At El Arish in Egypt, the quarantine doctor accompanied Raoul de Malherbe on horseback among the palm groves of the seashore, where he shot wild duck while his guardian looked on.[50] The gun would have been his own, as firearms were tolerated in most lazarettos. One detainee at Malta stood on his balcony for a few hours shooting at seagulls.[51] And at Smyrna, the theologian John Wilson was lucky enough to pass quarantine with friends in a rented cottage, where their 'principal exercise . . . consisted in musket and rifle practice'.[52] The existence of so much weaponry among travellers is no cause for surprise, as remote areas in the Levant and further east could be dangerous due to wild animals and brigands.

In a few places, those in quarantine needed only to listen to music to hasten the passage of time. Stendhal claimed that on Malta '*deux fois par jour on vient vous faire de la musique*', but it is not clear what he meant as no one else referred to it.[53] At Port Mahon in Minorca, the music came from a band of 14 musicians; these were local men who went aboard an American warship, apparently evading quarantine themselves. They imparted a 'cheering influence', playing 'with all the skill, spirit and animation for which the Balearic islands and Italy are so justly admired'.[54] It was, indeed, at Italy where serenading was practised most regularly, with Americans as the main beneficiaries. When Robert Semple was at Leghorn in 1806, he noticed a great animation around ships at quarantine within the mole:

> 'In some boats are musicians, who row under the sterns of vessels, especially those newly arrived, and play national airs, according to the flag which they see. Being under American colours, they were exceedingly noisy with 'Jefferson's March', and 'Yankee Doodle', until we dismissed them with a small piece of money. Other boats contained ballad-singers, who made the air resound with Italian ditties.'[55]

Eleven years later, little had changed, as Henry Matthews makes clear:

> 'As soon as we were safely moored within the harbour, a boat full of musicians made its appearance under the cabin-window, and we were serenaded with 'Rule Britannia', and 'God Save the King'. It is the custom to celebrate in this manner the arrival of every new comer, and to welcome him with the national airs of the country to which he belongs. A few hours afterwards, an American came to an anchor very near us, and we had then to listen to *Yankee Doodle's March*, with some other airs not at all tuneable to an English ear. This serenading is probably the remains of an old custom, when a voyage was considered an adventure of great danger, and the return of a ship an event worthy of extraordinary celebration.'[56]

A more cynical explanation would be that the serenaders were hoping to make an income from their captive audience. That would accord with the experience of the Revd Charles Swan in Naples Harbour, in 1824. He and his companions were entertained one morning by a couple of musicians who rowed out to the ship. They were outlandish and scruffy in costume and appearance; one of them played a bagpipe and the other a kind of reed. 'They obtained a few small pieces of money', noted Swan, 'and retired, doubtless well pleased with the power of their music'.[57] Busking of this kind was largely confined to the western Italian seaboard, because only there were travellers regularly detained for several days on board ship, either as a precursor of quarantine ashore or (less often) in lieu of it.

Sexual misbehaviour in quarantine would seem to have been well-nigh impossible, given the degree of supervision and the rules of non-physical contact. But that was not the impression given to Ida Pfeiffer at Aegina, when a servant girl was put into the same room as a bunch of steamer mechanics: 'after a few days the poor thing begged me for God's sake to take her into mine, as their behaviour towards her was extremely improper. What a situation would she have been in', mused Ida, 'had not a woman been accidentally among the passengers, or if I had refused her request!'[58] Elsewhere there was casual flirting. At Villa Franca, on the Italian-French border, it was just another way of killing the boredom: 'At this moment', wrote Nathaniel Willis,

> 'the Marseilles trader and the two Frenchmen are throwing stones at something that is floating out with the tide; the surgeon has dropped his Italian grammar to decide upon the best shot; the Belgian is fishing off the wall with a pin hook and a bit of cheese; and the two Sicilians are talking *lingua Franca* at the top of their voices to Carolina, the guardian's daughter, who stands coqueting on the pier just outside the limits.'[59]

At the Lisbon lazaretto in the 1860s, the flirting was more serious. The American John Ross Browne observed with interest the young Spanish wife of a wealthy black man from Mogadore being receptive to the advances of a young Parisian. The outcome might have been serious if the Frenchman had not been diverted by quarrels with a French-speaking Swiss.[60]

There must be other unrecorded instances of lazaretto romances, but nothing to compete with the story which follows.[61] The culprit was Casanova. If there was one environment in which the fabled philanderer would surely draw a blank, it would be a lazaretto. But not he. His wanderings took him to the lazaretto at Ancona in 1744, where he stalked the exercise yard throughout the day. Having spotted from his balcony a comely Greek slave, he dropped her a letter with certain instructions and persuaded his guardian not to lock him up after dark. The girl, at midnight, climbed on a bale which put her head almost at the level of a hole he had made in the floor of the balcony. With Casanova lying flat, there was some contact of arms against lips but little more. That was not enough for either of them. The girl succeeded in bulking up the goods she was standing on, and Casanova removed the nails from a plank in the balcony so as to make the aperture larger. The following night, the girl climbed up the baskets and bales, and this time her head and arms protruded through the hole in the floor. That was better, but still not enough. On the next night, Casanova managed to lift her through the floor of the balcony.

> 'I drew her up towards me, and my desires are on the point of being fulfilled. Suddenly I feel two hands upon my shoulders, and the voice of the keeper exclaims, 'What are you about?' I let my precious burden drop; she regains her chamber, and I, giving vent to my rage, throw myself flat on the floor of the balcony, and remain there without a movement, in spite of the shaking of the keeper whom I was sorely tempted to strangle.'

The next morning, the governor informed Casanova he was free to leave the lazaretto. The fact that he and the girl escaped with their lives can only be explained by the silence of the guardian, who must have feared for his own skin after such laxity of control.

Many travellers in a lazaretto overcame the boredom by carving their names or initials or otherwise writing on the walls. The British were inveterate gougers and did not hesitate to leave their mark even on ancient monuments. The Dunlop sisters visited Pompey's Pillar at Alexandria 'and found it of course traced all over with the illustrious signatures of Brown, Jones, and Robinson'.[62] As the Malta lazaretto was a great favourite of the British, the graffiti there was much in evidence as several travellers testify. George Waring observed that the soft stone walls of his 'prison . . . induced many of its inmates to carve their names, which are generally accompanied by the date and duration of their imprisonment'.[63] R.N. Hutton was more explicit:[64]

> 'A very favourite source of amusement to those who have performed quarantine [in Malta lazaretto] . . . appears to have been the very popular and peculiarly English failing of cutting out their names, and many must have taken considerable pains about their work, and have had a particular ambition to hand their names down to posterity by these means, for in many instances the letters are cut to the depth of half an inch in the stone. Some of these have verses or fragments attached; but the most curious is an epitaph, which has been carved with great care, and runs thus:
>
> TO THE MEMORY
>
> OF A
>
> QUARANTINE
>
> WHICH EXPIRED ON THE 15th AUGUST 1845
>
> AGED 14 DAYS
>
> LITTLE REGRETTED BY
>
> J C -----------'

Another witness to the Malta graffiti was the Comte de Salaberry, who found that the outer walls of his room in the Malta lazaretto were '*couverts de souvenirs de tous les genres*'.[65] These included mention that his room had once been occupied for 38 days by Baron de Weïssemberg. This inscription had been written by someone other than the Baron, and such memorials by proxy were also found elsewhere. At Marseilles, the room occupied by François Pouqueville bore mention of a former sojourn by the Duchess of Berry, which seems almost to have been a commemorative plaque.[66] As the decades passed, the enthusiasm for defacing surfaces did not. At Lisbon, in the 1860s:

> 'The walls were covered with the names of sundry poor fellows who had spent weeks, and even months, in this dreary prison, and who whiled away the time cutting out various fanciful devices and inscriptions, with the dates of their arrival and departure.'[67]

Many of these, of course, were Englishmen.

At least one defacement at Malta was politically charged. A wall at Fort Manoel, which acted as overspill accommodation for the lazaretto proper, had been decorated with the stars and stripes by some American visitors and captioned 'The Flag of Liberty'. But British inmates later drew a slave attached to the flagpole and a man standing over him with a whip.[68] Less contentious, but scarcely more acceptable, was the handiwork found in some of the lazarettos of Italy. At Ancona a saloon described 'as a lounging-place for the prisoners' was covered with writings and drawings by several nationalities. Most inscriptions were in Greek and Italian, followed by French and German. The British language came fifth. William Mure found these walls 'remarkable for little else than folly, dull sentimentality, or obscenity. In the latter [i.e. last] respect were more particularly distinguished those emanating from Italo-Greek authors'.[69] Peter Laurent had a similar experience further south at Barletta:

> 'The walls were covered with inscriptions in different languages; many French, Italian, and Greek travellers, seemed to have endeavoured to charm away their *ennui* by daubing the walls: names of Greek saints, terms of love in the French language, and those of obscenity in Italian, are seen in all parts of the building.'[70]

Occasionally, graffiti was devoted to poetry or philosophy. Some lines were terse or enigmatic, such as 'Life is the quarantine to eternity', which graced one of the rooms at Marseilles.[71] More often, however, it was doggerel of the kind Miss Pardoe found 'partially traced through the whitewash' at Orsova.[72] But erudition also found its niche. Edward Ives, in the lazaretto at Leghorn in 1758, found a Latin verse of 18 lines cut into a window shutter by its composer, an Irishman named William O'Carrol. Ives reproduced them in his book 'not for the goodness of the poetry, but because they sensibly struck me, as exactly corresponding with my own melancholy situation'.[73] Another classical scholar was William Turner, locked up at Trieste. Having noticed 'the numerous complaints scrawled on the walls by former imprisoned countrymen of mine', he wrote his own 'paraphrase of Horace's assertion of the possibility of being happy anywhere'.[74] Turner included the verses in his book.

On Sundays and other days of religious significance, travellers struggled to maintain their devotions. There was often a church or chapel attached to a lazaretto, but it was primarily for the funerals of those who died within the walls to minimize the risk of contagion by burial elsewhere. Nevertheless, there were sometimes facilities specifically for travellers in transit. At Cephalonia, there was a Greek church with a resident priest attached to the lazaretto, while at nearby Zante, monks of the Order of St Anthony maintained both a Roman Catholic church and a hospital.[75] There was also a Greek church attached to the Zante lazaretto.[76] At Trieste, seamen performing quarantine in their ships were allowed ashore every Sunday, under various precautions, to attend mass in the lazaretto chapel.[77] Nearby were separate burial grounds for Roman Catholics, Greeks and Protestants. The arrangement at Port Mahon on Minorca, when Britain had ceded the island to Spain, was more complicated. Adjacent to the lazaretto was an 'oratorio', which consisted of a circular range of secure rooms, each about 20 feet from a central pulpit surmounted by a flagpole. When the Spanish flag was hoisted, health officials conducted their charges to a designated room within the circle and the service commenced.[78] John Howard noted that the chapel at Genoa was in the middle of a row of apartments and had 'three sides open, that the elevation of the host may be seen in the opposite rooms'.[79]

On Malta, it was quite usual for English detainees to attend the chapel attached to Fort Manoel, as it had changed under British rule from Roman Catholic to a Protestant denomination. It was also normal for these services to be taken by Church of England clergymen who happened to be in detention. For Roman Catholics, however, there was no provision for mass either in Fort Manoel or in the lazaretto itself, and the devout were at some pains to accomplish their duties, as Samuel Bevan noted:

> 'Rising one day somewhat earlier than usual, I was surprised to observe a number of persons kneeling on the stones at the end of the open corridor, extending along the front of the building we occupied. As they simultaneously made the sign of the cross, and appeared all to direct their attention to one particular object, I soon discovered that their altar and officiating priest were at least a good half-mile off on the opposite shore. Waiting until the ceremony was over, I fetched my glass, and could then remark a small chapel in the side of the rock, wherein the service had been conducted, and from which the priest and a little crowd of devotees were now departing.'[80]

This little chapel was noted by other diarists, and indeed John Henry Newman was intrigued at the sight of 'a poor fellow in the Lazaretto close to us, cut off from the ordinances of his Church, saying his prayers towards the house of God which lay in his sights over the water'.[81] At Christmas, however, the authorities were more considerate towards Roman Catholics. Raoul de Malherbe, sharing his confinement with Monseigneur Collier, was happy that the latter was allowed the use of a little room for daily religious observance.[82]

For evangelical Christians, detention in a lazaretto was an opportunity. The missionary Robert Maxwell Macbrair arrived in Malta on a brig from Alexandria bound eventually for England. Some of the sailors were quarantined in adjoining rooms and allegedly indulged in 'drunken revels', although ribaldry was not an activity normally associated with detention at Malta. Macbrair 'admonished them of the evil of their ways; and when they were in a mood for such a purpose, I gave tracts respecting sin and intemperance'. One Irish sailor, son of a Protestant clergyman, came to Macbrair in great distress, reportedly sobbing at his own moral decadence and seeking 'instruction and prayer'. Unfortunately for the missionary, the sailor appeared to relapse before his release, but Macbrair was ever hopeful that one day 'the wanderer may reflect upon the instructions that he received in the lazaret'.[83]

Quakers in quarantine were in a unique position because their unusual attire attracted attention. There were confused views about their religious perspective. Stephen Grellet, an American, was almost a celebrity in the Marseilles lazaretto: 'Curiosity to see a Quaker frequently brings persons of various ranks and conditions to see and converse with me'.[84] Among these were Roman Catholic priests testing his spiritual commitment, followed by some Spaniards who thought that burning would not be too good for him. Even the captain of the lazaretto appeared 'desirous to obtain correct information, and often visits me on that account'. In fact, he was kept professionally busy, probably at the request of the authorities, comforting sick seamen and giving 'the cup of consolation' to an American woman dying of consumption.[85] Grellet was later detained in the lazaretto at Barletta, where his attire earned him visits from the town dignitaries, from others who were just curious and from priests eager for a constructive religious discussion.[86]

Grellet's sternest test came in 1832, when he travelled to Rotterdam from London with his fellow Quaker, William Allen. With the cholera pandemic gripping Europe, they were expecting the formality of a seven-day quarantine in Holland, but it proved to be an horrific ordeal. A sailor on board died of cholera, having drunk a large amount of cold water to cure a hangover. The terrifying implications of that were not helped by the 'rather appalling' sight of a doctor in 'a long black oiled silk gown, which reached to his feet, black gloves of the same material, and a black hood which covered his head and face, excepting the nose and eyes'. As the awfulness of his presence coincided with a thunderstorm, Allen and Grellet found comfort in their Bibles. Other deaths followed, even when the sick were allowed ashore, but the two Quakers were philosophical about their own fate and tireless in supporting others.[87]

Many travellers arrived at a lazaretto carrying letters and papers, sometimes for government, and most detainees created social correspondence during their stay. In Malta, letters for posting were received with tongs by 'the knight of the smoke of purification'.[88] Near Rostov-on-Don, as if tongs were not enough, papers were 'received by a man in tarred clothes and gloves'.[89] On arrival at Odessa, the traveller found that letters which had been sealed for posting were slit open and fumigated in boxes before dispatch.[90] Even if the traveller believed (as few did) that paper was a dangerous conveyor of disease, there was always the feeling that letters and dispatches were being opened for fumigation, despite being sealed, as an excuse to spy into the contents. That was the worry for Jean Dumont at Venice in 1691, when he fretted at being forced to surrender correspondence from a friend to a third party, 'so that I shall be oblig'd to deliver'em unseal'd to the Persons to whom they are directed'.[91] In 1838, the anticontagionist John Bowring used espionage as an argument for the abolition of quarantine restrictions. 'I was once admitted to a Lazzaret', he wrote, 'in the Austrian frontier – where I saw the correspondence of the East with England delivered to the authorities, every letter was opened, examined, fumigated – resealed and despatched'.[92]

There is no doubt that in border lazarettos, such as those on the Danube, letters were indeed read before resealing. The feckless director of the lazaretto at Calafat in Wallachia complained to James Skene that, although he met few travellers, 'the trouble of examining minutely into the circumstances of them, and of reading all the letters that cross the Danube, in order to send a detailed report to Bucharest, keeps me constantly occupied'.[93] But, the Danube aside, by the nineteenth century most lazarettos were too exercised by the volume of correspondence passing through their hands to worry about the contents, which were anyway of minimal interest. Most travellers were highly literate and had family and friends with whom they corresponded throughout their peregrinations. A steamer load of inmates to the lazaretto at Malta or Marseilles could produce a mailbag of paper, which the authorities, whether they liked it or not, were obliged to purify. There were two ways of doing this. At Marseilles, for instance, all letters were dipped in vinegar – the traditional method – and travellers were advised to have a correspondent in the port who would dry them before onward transmission.[94] The damage done by vinegar, both in smell and discolouration, encouraged most ports to use fumigation instead. At Malta in 1833, letters were

> 'laid on shelves in a sort of cupboard; a quantity of straw is then set on fire in a shallow iron pan, and the flame having subsided a little, a handful or two of composition, of which brimstone is the chief ingredient, is thrown over it, the pan is placed in the cupboard, and the doors are closed. In a few minutes the contents are considered to be sufficiently purified.'[95]

Every lazaretto had a component called a *parlatorio* where people in quarantine could converse with those in pratique. At Malta, John Henry Newman described it succinctly: 'It is a long naked building or barn, divided into several rooms, but intersected from one end to the other by two barriers parallel, breast high – between these guardians are stationed to hinder communication'.[96] In fact, there were three such places on the island. The second *parlatorio* was on shore on the Valletta side of the quarantine harbour, while the third was on the edge of the Grand Harbour. The larger of these two was the second *parlatorio*, 'a very long narrow building, divided into three parts by two walls running lengthways, and about six feet apart, so that the healthy and suspected parties have that space between them, which effectually prevents any contact'.[97] Guardians patrolled the middle, passing to those in quarantine goods bought from the 'healthy' side and supervising the payment of money in the other direction. Also on the healthy side were stationed errand boys, who took commissions for purchases and carried slates on which detainees could write a message for their friends at large.[98]

The system worked well, although detainees might find themselves 'somewhat embarrassed by bars and banisters', while others were amused that 'secrets of great import were necessarily confided in the loudest key'.[99] But the fact that the presumptive unclean and the assumed healthy were separated by such a small distance that the breath or odour of someone on one side could transmit without difficulty to the person opposite was a telling testimony to the doctrine of contagion. As long as the two sides could not actually touch, the proximity was deemed immaterial. Probably no *parlatorio* was used as much as the one at Odessa, where it became possible, and indeed normal, for ships to ride out their quarantine in the harbour. Their crews were allowed to land when they wished into a series of 'compartments' along one side of a quay, which were separated from the other side by wooden bars and wire mesh. There, all nationalities, in a babel of languages, transacted mercantile business or simply whiled away the boredom of their detention.[100]

In a few lazarettos the *parlatorio* was also a kind of supervised bazaar. The one at Malta had what Mary Carmichael called 'standing shops'.[101] Lucinda Griffith, in the same lazaretto, was intrigued by the nearness of buyer and seller, with only the rails as a barrier between them: 'Several articles of jewellery, of gold and silver filagree [*sic*]-work, and gloves and mittens, netted in black silk, all of native manufacture, were exposed for sale on one side of this bar'.[102] Money was paid into troughs of water and the goods passed over by long, iron tongs. R.N. Hutton found his purchases arrived on the end of a piece of wood. He characterized the produce as 'very fine gold and silver ornaments, silk mitts highly valued by English ladies, and flowers made of silver lace'.[103] The pantomime of payment through water amused many purchasers, among whom was Charles Terry, who looked at the hale buyer on the quarantine side and the 'dark, meagre, ill-favoured' vendor sitting in pratique and deduced that 'infection' was more probable in the latter.[104] Mary Carmichael reckoned that the quality of the filigree work equalled that of the workshops of Genoa, while the mittens were fine enough to be exported in their 'millions'.[105] For some travellers, however, the goods were tawdry. Albert Hervey dismissed them as 'Maltese crosses, chains, rings, and other articles of bijouterie; ladies mittens, canary birds, cakes, ices, and all sorts of trash'.[106]

The other lazaretto noted for its trading potential was Orsova, but the circumstances were different. The Austrians maintained a quarantine against the Wallachians to the north of the Danube and against the Serbs to the south, while the Wallachians had their own quarantine against the Serbs. But if the three nationalities could not intermingle, it was nevertheless necessary for them to trade, especially between Serbia and Wallachia. The result was a kind of *parlatorio* which was unashamedly a market and particularly useful to the Serbs and, therefore, the Turks, who crossed the river three times a week to do business there.[107] It was described as

> 'a long oblong shed, open all round, but roofed in. It is divided into three parts by wooden palings, and in the centre is another place partitioned,

> with a table in it for the quarantine and custom-house officers, who are on these occasions attended by an armed guard.'[108]

There were strict rules of conduct, with bargains struck through the quarantine guardians. Money was taken in tongs and immersed in a cup of vinegar, rather than water. Travellers reported 'a considerable traffic in pipe-heads, Turkish sweetmeats, fruits, ornaments, and other small articles', while the mixture of Oriental and European faces, clothes, languages and cultures made the spectacle a fascinating outpost where East met West.[109]

Travellers were only too aware that the purpose of quarantine was to allow time in which symptoms of plague might develop. There was always, therefore, a nagging concern that any illness arising during quarantine could extend the detention until the physician in charge felt able to state categorically that it was not plague-related. These fears were not helped by a comment in Murray's *Hand-Book* of 1840, which warned that 'the slightest indisposition in quarantine subjects the traveller to the suspicion of plague, and prolonged confinement'.[110] The evidence, however, would suggest that such worries were misconceived and that illness in quarantine was so commonplace that the authorities were seldom alarmed.

Murray's cautionary note appears to be based on attitudes which had been abandoned many years earlier. Thomas Dallam, arriving on Zante in around 1600, reported that quarantine from the Levant was normally ten days but, if any person was found sick on the last day, the period was doubled.[111] This fits with the warning of George Sandys, who visited Zante about ten years later, although he was unspecific about the extra period.[112] There is nothing, however, to suggest that this practice was widespread, and as the companions of Richard Chandler discovered, it was possible by 1766 to be feverish even in quarantine on Zante and still depart on time.[113] By definition, a lazaretto was an institution for the reception of people who might be ill, not a place where illness was abhorrent. This was especially so at Venice, while at Leghorn the second lazaretto was described in 1764 as '*un véritable hôpital de pestiférés*'.[114] There was, therefore, nothing incompatible between sickness and detention, and indeed there were many instances of persons suspected of plague, but not necessarily in quarantine, being admitted to a lazaretto for treatment. And when a traveller arrived chronically ill, it was not necessarily a question of remaining there indefinitely until he or she recovered or died. Princess Maria Theresa Asmar is a case in point. She arrived at Leghorn in 1832 in a miserable state:

> 'I was so shattered by the dreadful sickness to which I had been a martyr during almost the entire voyage, that I was extremely ill throughout the whole period of my confinement in the lazaretto; and when at length we were set at liberty, I was carried to a locanda in Leghorn, where I took to my bed, and remained there for three months in a most debilitated condition.'[115]

Attached to every lazaretto was a physician. Where the *spoglio* was practised, these men were routinely busy, but in most lazarettos they were there mainly to decide whether or not an illness was truly the plague, which reportedly they did very badly. John Bowring dismissed all native doctors in the Levant as incompetent, giving instances of them diagnosing plague from gangrene, syphilis, an abscess, a contusion, quinsy and delirium.[116] In fact, most doctors attached to lazarettos in the Levant were Europeans, typically French, Italians and Germans, but they were scarcely more highly regarded. John Davy called them (and quarantine directors) 'the weak part of the system'. He alleged that the doctors were poorly educated and came to Turkey 'as adventurers'.[117] Charles Monk, detained in the Hebron lazaretto, might have agreed with him:

> 'The doctor of the Quarantine, half French, half Italian, arrived this evening from Gaza, and paid me a very short visit, taking care to keep at a respectable distance. He is neither intelligent in his looks nor particularly engaging in his manners.'[118]

The Revd Justin Perkins, an American, understood that nearly 300 of these European doctors were in the Levant, and he accused them of being covert agents for the Vatican.[119]

Even in the West there was little confidence in quarantine doctors. Some caused dismay even by their appearance. HRH Mirza Abu Taleb Khan found himself at Genoa from the Levant in 1814.

> 'The physician who came aboard our ship was a meagre, sallow-looking person, who appeared as if just risen from the bed of sickness; whilst our crew were handsome healthy fellows. Having first looked at us, and then at himself, he seemed as if ashamed of the comparison, and, without examining our certificates, granted us permission to land.'[120]

Fifty years later, the doctor at Lisbon was no more inspiring:

> 'At noon the boat came, bearing in it a very sallow and cadaverous-looking gentleman, with very green gills and bilious eyes, and a great deal of brass on his cap and shoulders. . . . 'I am the physician of health', said the bilious man, in a very sickly voice.'[121]

And when doctors *were* more presentable, they were not necessarily any better. Julia Pardoe had no high regard for the doctor at Orsova:

> 'Twice each day we were visited by the medical officer, who just popped his head in at the door, and smiled forth: 'Ah! Quite well, quite well, I see – impossible to be better – good morning', and away he went, without affording us time to complain had we been so inclined.'[122]

The Rothenturn lazaretto had a German doctor who spoke no English, French or Italian. Frustrated by this failed communication, the Revd Robert Walsh reckoned the man must surely know Latin, in view of his training, 'but he could not comprehend or speak a word of it'. Walsh dismissed him as 'the most dull and ignorant perhaps of his profession'.[123] A more comical instance of language difficulty occurred at the Semlin lazaretto, where the doctor was also unacquainted with the main western tongues. The Italian companion of Francis Hervé was suffering badly from fleas or lice, but the doctor did not understand. Hervé and the Italian made graphic gestures to illustrate the problem, but their 'united dumb-show eloquence was exerted in vain'. Hervé, who was also a portrait painter, then had the brainwave of drawing 'a likeness of one of the insinuating little wretches from memory', by which the doctor 'was enlightened in an instant' and a treatment was prescribed – and worked.[124]

At the Malta lazaretto in the early days of British control, the doctors were army surgeons, but a Maltese physician was appointed to the Board of Health in 1826. Later, the doctors were Italian. Travellers usually found them most polite but not necessarily any use. In fact, Jean Jacques Ampère thought them '*la partie comique du drame*'.[125] He was quite seriously ill and almost too weak to move. Every morning one of the two doctors arrived at his door and, from a distance of ten feet, shouted 'show me your tongue!' They then asked questions, always the same ones, and prescribed drugs in which Ampère had no more confidence than he had in those prescribing them. He was careful to have the medicines ordered from town so as not to alienate the doctors who could have declared his illness contagious. But when their backs were turned, he threw his treatment in the sea.[126] Perhaps Hans Christian Andersen was tempted to do likewise in the Danube when he was locked up in the lazaretto at Orsova. All his party fell sick with stomach pains, and the doctor prescribed them a medicine 'excellent for Wallachian horses'.[127]

Among the litany of scorn and complaints, only one lazaretto doctor had a really good write-up. The Frenchman Raoul de Malherbe arrived at El Arish in Egypt in 1843 and struck up an immediate friendship with the camp physician, named Gian-Angelo de Dominis, a Venetian nobleman. This man, whom various setbacks had reduced to a life in the Levant, '*était un des hommes les plus aimables et les meilleurs que j'aie connus dans ma vie de voyageur*'.[128] But perhaps their joint duck-shooting sorties had something to do with the eulogy.

Conditions in some of the eastern lazarettos were so bad that many people thought them breeding grounds for disease. At Gumry in Armenia, the Revd Justin Perkins suffered a plague of flies, a sandstorm 'and a stench from animals that had died during quarantine, their bodies being left unburied'.[129] In a lazaretto near the Persian frontier, Captain Wilbraham 'found the sole accommodation for travellers consisted in some half-dozen subterranean cells, low and dark, and swarming with cockroaches'.[130] Another soldier, Captain Jesse, killed 180 'bugs' during his stay at Odessa, while Catherine Tobin found the fleas and mosquitos at Gaza were 'voraciously unmerciful'.[131] The Revd George Fisk spent a 'loathsome imprisonment' at Constantinople 'amidst rats, which gambolled about the room at night, and swarms of other vermin'.[132] But the western institutions, here and there, were not much better. John Murray, in his guidebook of 1840, warned of vermin in the lazarettos of Naples and Sicily, and a Frenchman at Malta regretted his nights spoilt by '*des hôtes malencontreux*'.[133]

Some lazarettos were inherently unhealthy by their situation, especially if surrounded by brackish water. James Minet heard of people who allegedly caught the plague when locked up at Santa Maura, but it was more probably malaria.[134] The lazaretto was terribly sited, 'surrounded as it is by salt lakes and stagnant marshes' and buzzing with mosquitoes, and detainees were invariably ill.[135] Nearby Zante was only marginally better 'adjacent to an undrained marsh', and William Turner believed he caught his 'delirious fever' there, although the authorities insisted otherwise.[136] Similarly, the lazarettos along the River Pruth were most unwholesome due to the marshy air, and the conditions might trigger an attack of fever or malaria for someone who had arrived in remission.

Even the lazaretto on Malta, healthily situated as it was, did not escape complaint. Lord Byron famously cursed it for a return of his 'Quotidian Tertian' caught in Greece; the building was too hot and the 'infernal oven' of a May sun put him 'in bad health & worse spirits'.[137] Joseph Bedlam thought 'he who has passed through such an ordeal of filth and annoyance [at Malta], without serious indisposition, may be safely permitted to go at large'.[138] But for every person who allegedly suffered on Malta, there were ten who found the climate and environment acceptable. It was the rodents which bothered some more than the heat and inevitable fleas. Mary Beswick, for instance, was happy enough at the lazaretto but suffered 'a bountiful supply of Rats', which forced her 'to stuff a Quilt under the Door to prevent them getting in'.[139]

A greater risk than fever in quarantine isolation was some kind of enteric disorder. Sufferers ascribed various causes. In 1758, Edward Ives entered quarantine at Leghorn and was immediately 'greatly distressed in my bowels, from a cold caught on board the vessel, and renewed the day we came to the Lazaretto'.[140] At Trieste, in 1806, Nicholas Biddle 'was a good deal indisposed owing to something I eat having disagreed with me, & from resuming my habits of eating after my fasts during the voyage'.[141] In 1827 Moses Montefiore, at the Malta lazaretto, arose one day 'with an attack of dysentery', which his wife reported to the superintendent of quarantine when he arrived on a social visit. He 'allayed all fears by informing me that this complaint had prevailed almost universally at Malta within the last week, but without creating the slightest degree of apprehension'.[142] John Bowring wrote scornfully in 1838 about the lazaretto at Beirut, where 'many had died of dysentery and other disorders, from which they were perfectly free when they entered'.[143] Charles Pridham was no more polite about conditions on the borders of Serbia. He entered a quarantine station 'in the enjoyment of perfect health; on quitting it, I was suffering from a severe cold and dysentery, occasioned by the barbarous neglect of the authorities to provide the first elements of comfort'.[144]

When a death occurred suddenly in a lazaretto, it was, as William Makepeace Thackeray put it, 'striking'.[145] In some places, the very approach to the building was a reminder of the fragility of life. At Orsova, for instance, the entrance passed through the graveyard of those who had died in detention. 'It was closely fenced', wrote Julia Pardoe, 'and rendered still more gloomy by a tall crucifix, painted red, and supporting a most revolting effigy of our Lord'.[146] Spirits at Orsova were not raised by the precise inventory of possessions always taken, as James Best discovered, 'to prevent robbery in case of the person dying in quarantine'.[147] Most lazarettos had a burial ground very near them, but they were usually more sensitively sited than the one at Orsova. The lazaretto at Trieste, thoughtfully, had 'small burying-grounds for those of each different religion'.[148]

A death was especially worrying for travellers who had teamed up with others or were lodged in adjoining rooms. For some of these people the worry was of a delayed release date; for others it was fear that a contagion was rife, in which case their days were possibly numbered. Thackeray could scarcely believe the death of a recent shipboard acquaintance.

> 'We were walking with him but two days ago on deck. One has a sketch of him, another his card, with the address written yesterday, and given with an invitation to come and see him at home in the country, where his children are looking for him. He is dead in a day, and buried in the walls of the prison.'[149]

Thackeray mentioned no diagnosis, which was not unusual with sudden deaths. And this uncertainty, together with the rapid decline of the patient, heightened the horror for those all around. Robert Snow, in the Malta lazaretto during 1841, noted in his diary that two of his 'fellow-prisoners' were ill and two priests had been called from Valletta. Two days later one of the sick men died, his companion was still dangerously ill and two more detainees were becoming unwell. 'In the afternoon', wrote Snow, as the body was laid out, 'we observed a large carrion crow hovering over the Fort, and finally over that part of the building in which the unfortunate man died'.[150] Not a good omen for the anxious.

Neither Thackeray nor Snow was as alarmed by a death as Lucinda Griffith. She and her husband had reached Malta from Alexandria on the steamer *India* and had become friendly with a Frenchman named Foudant. One day before their release, they learnt that he had suddenly died. 'I cannot describe the shock it gave me', wrote Mrs Griffith, 'to think that one I had known so short a time ago, full of health and spirits, should have been cut off so suddenly, and in such a fearful manner'.[151] In fact, she spent another page of her journal describing personal details of a hale and hearty Monsieur Foudant and trying to express her disbelief that he was dead. The Frenchman, it appeared, had been going to pay his quarantine costs when 'he suddenly fell back, and never spoke afterwards. His body, after death, was covered in blue spots'.[152] A hastily convened meeting of the board of health pronounced the death 'although not decidedly plague, to be very suspicious'. The 17 people who had shared quarantine quarters with Foudant were 'closely shut up for eighteen days longer'. But the prevailing rumour was that he had been poisoned from inhaling the odour of musk, of which he was storing a large quantity in his room, and indeed others claimed the smell had made them ill.[153]

Lucinda Griffith spent the next day 'low-spirited and poorly' and reached the nadir of her depression at the sight of an approaching line of open boats:[154]

> 'I turned to look at them, when to my horror I saw in the third, which was towed by the two first, a plain black coffin; it was placed across the boat, no pall covered it, but there it lay, bare and neglected, as if made up in haste and unconcern. Four guardians, who were appointed to bear it, sat on either side; two others followed in the next boat, and after a short interval another came in sight: this was occupied by a priest. Rivetted to the spot where I stood, I listened to the melancholy splash of the oars, and watched the mournful procession as it traversed the whole length of the harbour, until it was hid from view by the sharp angle of the lazaretto, as it shaped its course to the quarantine burial-ground, situated on the same island, and, although unseen, but a very few feet from us. And these were the remains of poor Monsieur Foudant. . . . I cannot fancy any thing more horrible than to breathe one's last in a lazaretto . . . where all disease is set down as the most terrible and contagious to which human nature is liable.'

It would have comforted Mrs Griffith to know that the scene she witnessed was so rare that no similar description has come to light, from Malta or elsewhere.

Notes

See general note as to references stated at the end of Chapter 1.

1 Giraudeau (1835, 395).
2 Sultana (1976, 68).
3 Monk (1851, ii, 152).
4 Hughes (1820, ii, 363); Pinkerton (1833, 131).
5 Carne (1830, ii, 323).
6 Montefiore (1836, 260).
7 Griffith (1845, i, 96–7).

8 Kinnear (1841, 307); Bevan (1849, 166).
9 D'Estourmel (1844, ii, 518, 525).
10 Walsh (1829, 311).
11 Ives (1773, 393–4).
12 Stent (1843, ii, 225); Heywood (1919, 41).
13 Carlisle (1854, 315).
14 Grosvenor (1842, ii, 292).
15 Montefiore (1836, 263).
16 Spencer (1837, i, 218).
17 Olin (1843, ii, 469–70).
18 Fitzclarence (1819, 487–8).
19 Kinnear (1841, 308).
20 Newman (c. 1961–2006, iii, 165, 189).
21 Stendhal (1932, ii, 404). He wrote 'Pignoti', but the allusion is to the polymath Lorenzo Pignotti.
22 Marchebeus (1839, 220); Slade (1840, 313).
23 Auldjo (1835, 240–1).
24 Giraudeau (1835, 395).
25 Macintosh (1854, ii, 78).
26 Walsh (1829, 312).
27 Heywood (1919, 49–52).
28 Bramsen (1820, ii, 125).
29 Ros (1855, 63).
30 Montefiore (1836, 261).
31 Auldjo (1835, 239–40).
32 Marchebeus (1839, 221).
33 Waring (1843, 59).
34 Ibid., 65.
35 Kinnear (1841, 307).
36 D'Estourmel (1844, ii, 521–2).
37 Holroyd (1839, 55–7).
38 *Hansard's Parliamentary Debates*, lxvi (London, 1842), 614.
39 Usborne (1840, 83).
40 Griffith (1845, i, 79).
41 Watson (1853, 78): 'Another great indulgence was the opportunity of making excursions about the harbour in the ship's boat, always, of course, under the yellow flag, and the watchful eye of a guardiano'.
42 Gadsby (1880, 541).
43 Young (1848, 442).
44 Hervey (1846, ii, 76–7).
45 Kinnear (1841, 307).
46 Waring (1843, 59).
47 Giraudeau (1835, 395–6).
48 Marchebeus (1839, 221).
49 Nerval (1851, i): '*Du reste, nous avions le droit . . . de nous baigner même dans la mer sous la surveillance d'un gardien*'.
50 Malherbe (1846, ii, 322).
51 Najaf (1839, i, 216).
52 Wilson (1847, ii, 422).
53 Stendhal (1932, ii, 398).
54 Woodruff (1831, 207).
55 Semple (1808, ii, 29).
56 Matthews (1820, 34).

57 Swan (1826, i, 36–7).
58 Pfeiffer (1851, 266).
59 Willis (1850, 10–11).
60 Browne (1867, 312–13).
61 Casanova (1958–60, i, 201–7), from which all of the following references are taken.
62 Dunlop and Dunlop (1858, ii, 237–8).
63 Waring (1843, 59).
64 Hutton (1847, ii, 313).
65 D'Irumberry (1799, 251).
66 Pouqueville (1821, v, 179).
67 Browne (1867, 313).
68 Gadsby (1880, 541n).
69 Mure (1842, ii, 308–9).
70 Laurent (1821, 258).
71 Laurent, loc. cit., who added 'the inscriptions of Barletta boast no such originality of thought'. He had not seen the Marseilles inscription himself, but it was the product of 'an Arabian hand'.
72 Pardoe (1854, 333).
73 Ives (1773, 399–400).
74 Turner (1820, iii, 332–3).
75 Panzac (1986, 157); Grasset (1800, iii, 51, 196).
76 Grasset (1800, iii, 196).
77 Turner (1820, 330).
78 Montague (1849, 86).
79 Howard (1791, 5).
80 Bevan (1849, 165).
81 Newman (c. 1961–2006, iii, 162).
82 Malherbe (1846, ii, 389).
83 Macbrair (1839, 193–4).
84 Grellet (1860, i, 113).
85 Ibid., 114.
86 Ibid., ii, 44–5.
87 Allen (1847, iii, 38–41).
88 Woodruff (1831, 45).
89 Reygang (1823, 255).
90 Slade (1840, 308).
91 Dumont (1705, 350).
92 Bowring (1838, 11–12).
93 Skene (1853, i, 272).
94 Plaisted (1757, 148). In the departmental archives at Marseilles, the stain and smell of vinegar among some quarantine papers can still make life difficult for a researcher.
95 Waring (1843, 58).
96 Newman (c. 1961–2006, iii, 162).
97 Waring (1843, 66).
98 Ibid.
99 Woodruff (1831, 46); Bevan (1849, 165).
100 Brooks (1854, 30–1).
101 Montauban (1846, 12).
102 Griffith (1845, i, 80).
103 Hutton (1847, ii, 310).
104 Terry (1848, 97).

105 Montauban (1846, 12).
106 Hervey (1846, ii, 75).
107 Snow (1842, 32); Elliott (1838, i, 132); Marmier (1846, i, 261–2).
108 Monson (1840, 145).
109 Paget (1839, ii, 125).
110 Murray (1840, 217–18).
111 Dallam (1893, 89).
112 Purchas (1905, 92).
113 Chandler (1817, ii, 336).
114 Grosley (1770, iv, 19).
115 Asmar (1844, ii, 263).
116 Bowring (1838, 14).
117 Davy (1842, ii, 452).
118 Monk (1851, ii, 144).
119 Perkins (1843, 486).
120 Abu Taleb Khan (1814, ii, 290).
121 Browne (1867, 305).
122 Pardoe (1854, 333).
123 Walsh (1829, 304).
124 Hervé (1837, ii, 326–7).
125 Ampère (1868, 526–7).
126 Ibid.
127 Andersen (1846, iii, 175).
128 Malherbe (1846, ii, 315).
129 Perkins (1843, 124); most lazarettos had separate facilities for the quarantine of cattle and horses.
130 Wilbraham (1839, 74).
131 Jesse (1841, i, 60); Tobin (1855, 241).
132 Fisk (1844, 419).
133 Murray (1840, x); Marchebeus (1839, 221).
134 Minet (1958, 253).
135 Spencer (1851, ii, 215).
136 Turner (1820, i, 172).
137 Byron (1973–82, ii, 44).
138 Beldam (1851, ii, 303).
139 Beswick (1997, 35).
140 Ives (1773, 395).
141 Biddle (1993, 207).
142 Montefiore (1836, 262).
143 Bowring (1838, 13).
144 Pridham (1851, 146).
145 Thackeray (1846, 63).
146 Pardoe (1854, 333).
147 Best (1842, 321).
148 Turner (1820, iii, 330).
149 Thackeray (1846, 63).
150 Snow (1842, 78).
151 Griffith (1845, i, 88).
152 Ibid., 89.
153 Ibid.
154 Ibid., 89–90, 92.

5 Reckoning and departure

The overriding sensation for detainees in a lazaretto was that of serving a prison sentence when they had done nothing wrong. Indeed, for many travellers there was no suggestion that they might even pose a significant risk. Yet if they baulked at the system, they did so at their peril. If quarantine was not a prison sentence, it was but one step away, and recalcitrance was as dangerous for a traveller as it would be for a convict. Bartholomew Plaisted in 1750 advised: 'it will be much the safest Way to comply with the establish'd Rules in every Thing', and of course most people did.[1] But the threat of a reprisal did not prevent some travellers from trying to evade quarantine and others from refusing to do as they were told.

Evasion of quarantine was rarely practised in the western Mediterranean because most travellers arrived by sea, and the opportunity to slip away between ship and shore was rare indeed. But with the connivance of other parties it was not impossible. Arriving at Malta in 1610, George Sandys sensibly disregarded dangerous advice. He had been deposited on the shoreline in the Grand Harbour of Valletta by a ship which continued its voyage. The health boat directed him to the overhang of a rock where he might spend the night before being taken to the lazaretto in the morning. Sandys had no provisions, and the 'ribald' French crew of a passing felucca urged him to enter the town and return before daybreak.[2] By deciding to stay where he was, he probably saved his own life.

Patrick Brydone and his party had a different, but no less serious, problem at Messina. They were sitting in the harbour in their small vessel, admiring the view, when they realized that the name of one of their servants had been omitted from the bill of health. As the health boat was arriving, there was a moment of panic: they bundled the man into a hammock and stowed him below. He was forced to stay there virtually all day as the health officials and consuls tarried on board. As the days passed, Brydone and the ship's master (who had the most to lose) became increasingly anxious. Every time they ventured ashore they seemed to bump into someone from the health office, and all the time the servant led a mummified existence below the hatches: 'for if he be discovered', admitted Brydone, 'we shall probably get into a very bad scrape'.[3] Indeed, they would have done.

DOI: 10.4324/9781003195733-6

Further east, deliberate evasion was widespread. This was partly because some journeys were overland, but even arrival by sea presented illegal opportunities. On Zante, in 1795, the British consul had no scruples about smuggling English tourists into his villa.[4] Elsewhere, loose procedures, imperfectly marked borders, badly policed byways and a sufficient bribe made it possible to avoid quarantine stations altogether, especially when the traveller was accompanied by a knowledgeable local. In one example of 1804, Sir William Gell landed on the Greek island of Samos from Asia Minor at a time of plague. He was heading for the island's main town, but at the first village some health guardians blocked his route. It mattered little. 'As to the immorality of eluding the sham quarantine in . . . Greece', wrote Gell, 'I think the most squeamish conscience might be easy under the crime'. He conversed with the guardians, who had

> 'the kindness most politely to show us a circuitous path by which to avoid the village, handed us, with great urbanity, over the garden walls and through the hedges . . . [and] received our money at several different times . . . in the perfect conviction they were performing essential service to their country.'[5]

More than 60 years later, Mark Twain was even more cavalier about Greek quarantine and needed no connivance among the locals. His ship arrived at Piraeus from where the tourists on board expected to visit Athens. But a quarantine against cholera meant the vessel and all aboard had to remain 11 days in the harbour. The captain thought this excessive and resolved to steam on to Constantinople after an overnight stay to refresh supplies. Twain and three others conspired to slip ashore and make for the Acropolis during this brief delay. They reached their objective, but the return journey was complicated by vineyard owners who accused them of stealing grapes. They managed to reach the steamer, which had lowered a boat to pick them up, but the health officials were cruising offshore and they narrowly missed arrest and certain imprisonment.[6]

For every traveller who evaded quarantine, there were another two who were simply rebellious. The practice of resisting or confronting officials, however offensive or incompetent their attitude, was never sensible, as the German Julius van Klaproth discovered near Tiflis in 1807. He was an influential diplomat and academic travelling with an impressive escort, but they were no match for the local commandant of the fortress, who also controlled the quarantine station. At first, all was serene and when they arrived in the evening the commandant came down to meet them. 'He was, as is usual with him, much inebriated', noted von Klaproth, 'but nevertheless took several glasses of punch with us'. He then promised to send fresh horses and an escort in the morning for the rest of their journey. When these failed to arrive, messages were sent to the fort to question the delay. Eventually, in the evening, the commandant arrived with the horses, but it was then too dark and dangerous to set off. A Russian major accompanying von Klaproth 'remonstrated inoffensively' with the commandant who went away without a word, leaving an instruction that if they did not wish to leave that night, they had to remain three days in quarantine as a kind of fine. And so they had. This was all the more galling for von Klaproth as the quarantine was 'absolutely unnecessary, as no part of the baggage of travellers is aired, and they themselves are not subjected to any examination; for which indeed the inebriated officers cannot spare time'.[7]

In earlier years, especially in Venice, it was more dangerous to attack the system, and by implication the government, than it was to be rude to individuals. In failing to understand this in 1691, Jean Dumont nearly came to grief. He had arrived in Venice aboard a merchantman in the knowledge that his 40 days of quarantine would begin only when he left the ship. But a commercial dispute delayed landing by four days, which would not be deducted from the quarantine. Dumont was livid. He confessed to being 'naturally of too free a Humour' and expressed his 'Impatience and Indignation in very bold and emphatic Terms'. It then dawned on him that everyone else was keeping quiet and looking embarrassed. The ship's master took him to one side, explaining he was 'ruin'd' for having spoken out against the authorities as the guardian was 'certainly an Informer'. What really worried Dumont was the master's next comment: that he would never have been so forthright for a hundred thousand crowns, adding some 'Tragical Stories' about those who had lost their lives for less. Your only chance, said the master, is to bribe the guardian to keep quiet. So Dumont gave him two sequins and grovelled for the man's favour. In fact, the guardian did inform against him, but perhaps not as forcefully as he might have done. The inquisitor sent a note to the prior of the lazaretto about the 'very turbulent and impatient Frenchman' in his custody, but the reprimand went no further.[8]

That experience contrasts with the much later detention of the American John Ross Browne in the lazaretto of Lisbon. The passing of two and a half centuries meant that the authorities were now fair game for criticism, and indeed in few other places would they have been as touchy as in Venice. The problem for Browne and his co-travellers was that they were not expecting any quarantine at all, but their appeal on these grounds was rejected. If Browne himself was phlegmatic, two of his companions were not:

> 'When the Portuguese official announced to us that we must still serve five days, the young Parisian danced with rage, tore his hair, called upon all the heavenly powers to give him patience to endure this outrage, and wound up by pronouncing the Portuguese government a brutish and villainous concern. He was followed by a Swiss Frenchman, who became still more excited; clenched his fist and shook it in the officer's face.'[9]

But nobody seemed to mind.

Sometimes the subject of a dispute was not revealed, as in the case of James Minet at Orsova. He was not a militant man but he fell out with the director of the lazaretto, who threatened him with ten days in prison. Minet mused that it was the 'first occasion I have found myself in hot water for a very long time past', so it can be deduced that his grievance had some substance.[10] Certainly, the British generally were not afraid of confronting what many deemed tinpot bureaucracy which had little to do with public health. Eliot Warburton became angry at Kartal, near Constantinople, when he was expected to add days to his own quarantine to match those of certain Persian princes with whom he had been travelling and who 'were under surveillance'. He complained to the director and was ordered to await the sultan's pleasure. But Eliot retorted

> 'that, having fulfilled all the quarantine requirements, I should wait for no permission, but walk out, and he [the director] might tell his sentry to fire upon a British subject if he dared. . . . The sentry stopped me; I shouted at him the only Turkish word I knew – pushed unceremoniously past him – and found myself upon the sea-shore.'[11]

He had got away with it.

The British on yachts were especially belligerent. Arriving at Syra in 1840, Lord Londonderry and his party were told they had to wait 14 days for pratique, and 'two dirty Greek guardians' were placed on the yacht. But at this 'the gentlemen rebelled', the guardians were sent packing, and 'setting the Greek authorities at defiance' the yacht sailed on to British-controlled Corfu.[12] Another aristocrat, the 1st Duke of Buckingham and Chandos, had a torrid time at Girgenti in Sicily in 1828. Pratique was initially granted, but then rescinded because the names of the crew were on the passport rather than the bill of health. Buckingham was led to believe the problem could be solved if his various papers were sent to the *Intendente*, who worked from the town rather than the harbour. After waiting for many hours and hearing nothing, Buckingham sent a boat ashore. Four hours later, there was still no news and the boat had not returned. Buckingham then sent another boat, with armed 'marines' to investigate. They discovered the first boat under arrest and guarded by a sentry. At the sight of the marines, the Sicilians were prepared to compromise, and a soldier arrived with a message from the *Intendente* indicating that pratique was possible. The messenger was holding the original papers, which Buckingham's men then requested. No, came the answer, not until all expenses attaching to pratique had been satisfied. So the soldier was then rushed and the papers retrieved by force. Buckingham then considered the matter settled although it had taken 12 hours. The next morning he sent a boat back into the harbour to buy provisions and deliver a letter of complaint destined for the King of Naples and his Viceroy in Sicily. But the health office had the last word as the letter was refused and kicked back into the boat.[13]

The threat of violence at Girgenti was echoed a few years later at Augusta, also in Sicily. Captain Roberts, on Byron's former yacht *Floridiana*, sought permission from the health office to buy provisions which needed only to be collected from the water's edge. But the officials wanted full fees for pratique, as well as the disembarkation of all those on the yacht. Captain Roberts then threatened to sail on immediately.

> 'At this prospect of losing their prey they became furious, and said that if we dared to act in that manner they would send gun-boats in pursuit, which would fire into us. We laughed, and telling them we were well-provided with excellent rifles, said we should wait for the gun-boats outside the harbour. We then sailed unmolested by pursuit.'[14]

In the instances just given, there were elements of bluff and bluster on the part of the authorities, and no shots were fired in anger by either side. But how real was the risk? Warburton and the yachtsmen had all taken the gamble that whatever the local rules, no foreign institution would risk the wrath of Britain by killing or wounding its citizens. Other travellers, however, were by no means so confident in the protection of their passports, as their writings testify. Alexander Kinglake gave the most chilling and eloquent warning:

> 'If you dare to break the laws of the quarantine, you will be tried with military haste; the court will scream out your sentence to you from a tribunal some fifty yards off; the priest, instead of gently whispering to you the sweet hopes of religion, will console you at duelling distance, and after that you will find yourself carefully shot, and carelessly buried in the grounds of the Lazaretto.'[15]

Kinglake was near the Danube at the time, but the warnings were universal. At Zante, George Sandys urged compliance, 'it being death to him that shall come ashoare [*sic*] without licence'.[16]

At Otranto, Samuel Evers was shocked and frightened: 'so severe are their laws against a breach of the rules of quarantine, that any person so offending, is liable to be put to death by the first person who meets him'.[17] Merideth Johnes, referring to the Beirut lazaretto, likened the inmates to prisoners of war, 'or something like it, seeing that, should any one attempt to break out, the soldiers on guard would shoot him down without the least ceremony!'[18] Ironically, in the eyes of a visitor from the Middle East, where the death penalty was never exceptional, the severity of quarantine caused some surprise. HRH Najaf Koolee Meerza, in quarantine at Malta, remarked (in a rather quaint translation from the Persian): 'The law of the Franks does not inflict death as a common punishment, but punishments are either fines, imprisonment, or banishment; yet the sin of breaking the quarantine is condemned as crimes to death'.[19]

Despite these apocalyptic warnings, there appears to be no evidence that any western traveller, let alone any Briton, was shot for quarantine disobedience. Such executions as there were, are recounted by travellers as hearsay. Adolphus Slade recounted the fitful introduction of quarantine at Constantinople, where it could be strictly enforced one minute and dispensed with the next. He learnt this had caught out a Jew who arrived on the steamer from Smyrna and, 'either heedless or ignorant of the existence of quarantine', landed immediately as he had always done. 'He was taken up and shot'.[20] This barbarity made no sense, because an hour later the rest of the passengers were allowed ashore without restriction. Slade then went on to Odessa, where he heard 'that a man had been recently shot *sans ceremonie* for having gone outside the limits' of the lazaretto.[21] Surprisingly, the most poignant incident took place on Malta. Jean Giraudeau recounted the fate of a local man in quarantine from Tunis, who tried to row ashore at midnight on learning that his son was dangerously ill. Unfortunately he was seen, shot and seriously injured. His wife was called and embraced him, which consigned her in turn to the lazaretto, where she soon learnt of the deaths of both her husband and son.[22]

This story, if correct, does little credit to the reputation of the British at the main lazaretto in the Mediterranean for which they were responsible. On the evidence, however, of other travellers, the guardians on Malta were not as trigger-happy as they were elsewhere. Giraudeau's anecdote arose in the context of his own recreational boat trip, when he was advised not to go too close to the shore as the sentries would open fire at any attempt to disembark. In fact, as has been shown previously, it was sometimes possible to land at certain remote beaches as long as the guardian aboard approved, but more to the point the sentries at Malta did not seek to kill or even wound with an opening shot. Joseph Strutt discovered this for himself in 1821. He had been breaking off specimen pieces of stone at the edge of the quarantine harbour (which was allowable), but then entered the water to wash his hands. A sentry immediately fired at him, which made Strutt most indignant. But he learnt later that, except around the lazaretto itself, their muskets were loaded with blanks. The first shot was always no more than a warning, although any other shots would be with a live round.[23]

There is as much evidence of harsh treatment by the health authorities of their own guardians as of their detainees. The memoirs of the Revd Justin Perkins, an American missionary, provide a graphic tale of brutality. Perkins was not squeamish, but he was disgusted by the discipline at the quarantine station of Gumry on the border of Armenia. Passing time in his tent (as there was no lazaretto building), he had been aware of 'constant wrangling' in the health office, and the disputes invariably ended in somebody being beaten. He was appalled

> 'that scarcely a day passed without bringing with it instances of flogging . . . and some of them, I should judge, must have been well-nigh

> mortal. Never before was I so heart-sickened with the rule of brutal force. Every little quarantine irregularity, without judge or jury, seemed to incur the rigor of the lash or club from a boorish Russian, or oftener from some other *civilized* European in the Russian service.'[24]

This was by no means the only instance of flogging within a quarantine station. At Odessa, Lord de Ros dismissed his waiter for being too dirty and promoted a lamplighter (at the man's entreaty) to the same position. It transpired that this new waiter was actually a thief, who soon absconded. His punishment, when caught, would be a flogging followed by conscription into the army and a posting to the Caucasus. The dirty waiter could expect a flogging as well for being negligent.[25] Also at Odessa, Lieutenant-Colonel Stuart related, with no obvious sentiment of shame, that a member of his party 'played a trick' on a guardian by falsely reporting that his roommate was ill. For not reporting this himself, even though the illness was untrue, the guardian 'was liable to receive eighty blows' while the prankster went unpunished.[26]

Flogging of corrupt employees was also practised on Zante when the island was administered by Britain. Consul Foresti sent an elderly servant to William Turner to ease his detention; at first the man seemed to do a satisfactory job at cooking and housekeeping. But Turner soon discovered that he was being 'unconscionably' robbed. When the servant was detected, he was

> 'flogged round the island, by order of General Campbell, who would have been justified by law in hanging him, for the offence that entailed his punishment, viz., delivering stolen articles to an accomplice out of the lazaretto, by which he might have introduced the plague to the island.'[27]

Casanova, single-minded as he was, could not bear a grudge against his guardian for stopping him jumping down to the courtyard below to meet a young slave girl, as the man's 'life might have been the penalty'.[28] But only one instance has come to light of a quarantine official being executed (or at least sentenced to execution) for negligence. This was at Alexandria in 1802, where William Wittman noted that 'one of the centinels [*sic*], a Sepoy, was tried by a court-martial and sentenced to be shot, for having suffered two Arab prisoners to make their escape from quarantine'.[29]

It may seem remarkable, given the boredom and uncompromising rigidity of quarantine, that some travellers actually enjoyed it. For some, the enforced delay could be a haven of calm after tiring explorations and a dangerous voyage. It was, as John Morritt declared at Barletta, a chance to be 'perfectly re-established'.[30] Constantine Tischendorff, detained for a fortnight at Syra, had a more philosophical view:

> 'Although the idea of quarantine is in itself disagreeable, yet did this period – may I call it a truce? – appear to form an essential link in the

> chain of the incidents of my journey . . . this spiritual collecting of the mind, this repose of quarantine, was very desirable.'[31]

Repose was indeed the word on many people's lips. Again at Syra, Eliot Warburton expressed his ambivalence: 'At length our quarantine is finished; I almost regretted our release, for the perfect repose that it necessitated was very grateful after incessant and laborious travel'.[32] At Marseilles, Anatoly Demidoff was pleased 'to seek in the lazaretto an interval of repose and solitude, charmed by many a reminiscence'.[33] Also at Marseilles, the Count de Forbin welcomed 'an opportunity to court a repose that I stood in need of . . . and I could feel myself in almost agreeable circumstances'.[34] Sarah Lushington found a similar prospect at Malta:

> 'I had led such a wandering and fatiguing life for some time past, and been so harassed by the tempestuous weather of the Mediterranean, that the tranquillity of the confinement was as agreeable to my feelings, as it was beneficial to my health.'[35]

There was also a need to adjust from the customs and habits of the East to what was considered the relative sophistication of western ways. It was in this light that Henry Rooke assessed his quarantine at Leghorn in 1782: 'I submit patiently to my captivity, since it is a condition annexed to my arrival in Europe, happy to have exchanged the barbarous climes of Asia and Africa, for regions of taste, pleasure and refinement'.[36] Sensibilities aside, detention could be acceptable in almost any lazaretto if the weather was not too hot or too cold, if the company was tolerable and if beds and food were no worse than expected. As Lieutenant-Colonel Stuart observed at Odessa: 'It is all a mistake to think that a lazaretto must be an unpleasant place, or that time must hang heavy on one's hands therein'.[37]

The lazaretto which received the highest praise was (as usual) Malta. In a spell of lovely summer weather, the view was at its best. Joseph Sherer watched the ships arriving with Sicilian fruits or the 'pretty red cattle of Barbary', smiled at 'the gambols of swimmers and divers', and was soothed at sunset by 'the hymns or songs of the mariners'. It was unsurprising, therefore, that he 'could not but be thankful and contented'.[38] George Waring felt he 'could be very happy in this place for a much longer time than we have spent in it, especially if many of one family were here together'.[39] John Auldjo went even further:

> 'The lazzaretto is a little world within itself, highly interesting for many reasons; and I confess I felt rather sorry as the time approached when we were to quit our quiet, tranquil abode, and be again let loose upon the busy, noisy world.'[40]

Even the fault-finding Lucinda Griffith left the Malta lazaretto with a tinge of sadness: 'Now we are really free, we feel almost sorry that we are going to leave, and, I dare say, we shall often look back to our quiet life with regret'.[41] Moses Montefiore went even further. He and his wife had endured a night-long storm so severe on the approach to Malta, that all aboard, including the master, had feared the ship might founder. In fact, so traumatic had it been that Montefiore, on the anniversary of that night during the rest of his life, reread the biblical verses he had entered in his diary when death seemed highly likely. When they eventually made the quarantine harbour, the relief made them ecstatic. It was therefore not surprising that quarantine to them was more than a chance to recuperate, and Montefiore 'was so comfortable as to wish they would prolong the term of quarantine, in lieu of shortening it'.[42]

Trieste was not far behind for satisfied inmates. William Turner, in 1817, was only too glad to be there: 'My feelings in quarantine were very different from those of the other prisoners, who were all grumbling and discontented, while I was quite contented and happy, having been so long accustomed to the want of comfort'. Turner summarized the secret of his satisfaction as 'a good bed, a good fire, a good room, occupation, health, good tobacco, and a Turkish pipe'.[43] Certainly, Trieste had more travellers satisfied than not. Twenty years later, no one in the group which included T.H. Usborne had a bad word to say about it. He found 'our time passed so quickly and agreeably, that there was not one of our party that was not sorry when the day arrived which gave us pratique'.[44] And at Trieste in 1840, George Scharf and his companions were 'all very sociable and merry . . . and the time passes happily on'.[45] Sociability was indeed the key to a happy detention, even in the lazarettos along the Danube. At Orsova, Captain Best found himself compulsorily 'chummed' with three other young bloods, two of them military men like himself and the third a personable American. They had the time of their lives. 'Certainly', Best declared, 'never were there stowed together in a lazaretto four persons who agreed better than we did', and his euphoria extended to the guardian: 'a most willing, excellent fellow, and a capital servant'.[46] Not many travellers wrote like that.

Even in the Levant, where people could be caustic about conditions, it was possible to find contentment for the same reasons of relief, repose and recuperation which applied in the West. Catherine Tobin confessed,

> 'Strange as it may seem, we could not quit the lazzaretto at Gaza without *some* feelings of regret. We had enjoyed three days' rest from the fatigue of constant travelling, and found abundance of occupation to prevent the time from hanging heavily on our hands.'[47]

At Beirut, Gérard de Nerval had some complaints, but the view was breathtaking and the seashore a constant delight: '*Une fois familiarisé avec ce lieu sauvage et maritime, j'en trouvai le séjour charmant*'.[48] And in case the French temperament may be thought an inherent advantage, there is the testimony of the Revd Henry Formby in Palestine that, 'even an Englishman may be very happy in quarantine, if he will'.[49]

When quarantine was over, the bills for lodging and sustenance, including the wages of the guardians, were settled with varying degrees of reluctance. The Austrians claimed that the lazaretto at Semlin was run at government expense for the convenience of travellers, but as Francis Hervé discovered, 'if you take quarters under any thing in the shape of a roof, you must pay for it, and that pretty handsomely'.[50] Indeed, Murray's handbook of 1840 warned that costs at Semlin were 'exorbitant'.[51] The Revd Robert Walsh was disenchanted with the costs at Rothenturn, also in Austria:

> 'Last came the different persons to be paid their bills, one charging what I thought unreasonable, for poor meat and sour wine; and another asking four paper florins, nearly a silver dollar, per night, for a pallet stuffed with straw, or flock. . . . I threatened to complain to the Governor of Hermanstadt of all this, – but so does every one else, and I was disregarded.'[52]

As regards expenses at all lazarettos, whether for food or accommodation, travellers' comments were predictably mixed. Edmund Spencer thought charges for provisions at Galatz 'would have been less at the London Hotel at Vienna, so famous for the excellence of its appointments', while at Aegina the list of charges was so long and severe that some inmates could not afford a hot meal and 'lived the whole twelve days on bread, cheese, and dried figs'.[53] But most people found costs, especially in the Levant, to be quite moderate. At Alexandria, in 1842, a figure of three piastres a day for board was called 'very trifling' by Ida Pfeiffer, while at Hebron in 1848 Charles Monk was given a bill nearly two-thirds lower than he had been led to expect.[54] In Greece, the lazaretto at Piraeus charged seven drachmas a day (five shillings) for a first-class bedroom, five drachmas (three shillings and sixpence) for a second-class one and three drachmas (two shillings) for a sitting room.[55]

Exact figures are sometimes quoted by travellers for one part or another of their quarantine expenses, but they are usually in local currency and mean little. At the Malta lazaretto in the 1840s, detainees were advised that the total costs 'for living, furniture, guardians, one servant, a washerwoman during the whole time (which is unnecessary), letters, coffee, fruit, and other extras for lunch or supper, for one person is about 11*l*. 10*s*., *without wine*'. These costs fell to about £9 a day each for two people sharing and to as little as £6 apiece for a group.[56] In fact, it could be a lot cheaper if some of the frills were dispensed with. Henry Fane spent 14 days in the Malta lazaretto in 1840 in a party of five, and it cost him only 18 guineas, which was roughly the cost of his steamer ticket from Gibraltar to Falmouth.[57] Two travellers from different social ranks have left very detailed accounts of their quarantine costs. The 6th Duke of Bedford and his entourage spent, over 20 days, just over 4,000 *livres* for a wide array of services including three washerwomen and two kitchen hands, which was the equivalent of £153 10s in sterling.[58] This figure may be compared with the costs of Francis Galton in the lazaretto at Syra, published by Enid Slatter, where a ten-day detention in 1840 cost him around 55 drachmas or a little more than £2 at the exchange rate then in force.[59] Hidden expenses arose in some lazarettos, where guardians and others might be susceptible to a bribe, and in many it was usual to tip. When Bartholomew Plaisted left the lazaretto at Marseilles, he paid three *livres* each to his guardian, the man who conducted his fumigation, the gate porter, the waitresses in the 'Eating House' and the woman who brought him his post.[60]

The medical formalities of departure (usually on the day preceding the scheduled release) bothered, intrigued or even amused the diarists. In many lazarettos the process of checking for signs of plague was reminiscent of the inspection on arrival. At Syra, the physician asked Sir Moses and Lady Montefiore to feel their own armpits 'and other parts of the body'.[61] Ida Pfeiffer experienced something very similar at Alexandria, where the physician was an old man 'with a spy-glass in one hand and a stick in the other'. Everyone had to strike themselves on the chest and in the side, the women being led to a separate room by 'a great female dragon'.[62] At Otranto the physician did a little more than observe, feeling the travellers' armpits for himself and then checking their pulse rate.[63] At Gaza, Dr. Eperon asked in French if people were well. With the answer in the affirmative, he would express his satisfaction but insisted on a show of tongues.[64] At Syra, the medical officer adopted a stern face when asking those departing to strike their armpits and groins. But when no evidence of pain creased their faces, 'he put on a most friendly and courteous smile' and stepped forward to shake each person's hand.[65]

The authorities at Malta were relatively relaxed at departure time. George Waring noted that the physician 'asked one question only, "Gentlemen, are you in good health?" which being answered in the affirmative, he made a low bow and took his leave'.[66] Had they had notice of his visit, Waring and his companions would have demonstrated their fitness by playing a game of tennis, although the location for that was not explained. John Auldjo, also at Malta, was similarly amused that the doctor addressed everyone with a trite form of words. This time, it was 'Pretty well? – ah! I see, quite well'.[67] Captain Best found even less formality at Orsova, where 'the little doctor of the establishment . . . announced to us our free pratique by shaking hands with each'.[68]

Odessa, predictably, took matters more seriously. In 1839, apart from the usual striking of armpits in the presence of a male or female official, a Lutheran priest made those departing swear an oath that no items had been concealed during quarantine.[69] A few years later the priest was Roman

Catholic, which caused Charles Terry to observe, 'I suppose Protestant parsons are scarce, as I got away without any clerical visitor'.[70] Terry was lucky to escape the formality, as Adolphus Slade found the oath was taken 'with all the forms of religion, regarding our health, and non-communication with other parties'. Slade's group had a choice of priests and opted for a Russian one. In the event, there were three of them:

> 'A box, with a glass lid, containing saints' images and relics, was placed before us on a table. The chief priest then robed himself, and recited a long string of sentences, utterly unintelligible to those to whom they were addressed; while each of us held up our forefinger (by order), and nodded occasionally, as if in assent. The ceremony terminated by our kissing the glass cover; and we were then declared to be purified in mind and body.'[71]

Slade was lucky because a Jew was leaving the lazaretto at the same time with a suspicious boil which the examining doctor failed to notice.

The greatest rigmarole for release occurred at one of the worst and least frequented lazarettos. This was Rothenturn, as the Revd Robert Walsh recounted:

> 'The Doctor came by candle-light in the morning; his man brought a pan of charcoal, on which he threw a few pinches of nitre; he then walked round me in a circle, like a magician, and so I was purified. The Inspector came and looked at my clothes, where my dirty linen, &c., lay in a heap on the floor, as I had brought it from the plague district; and in that state it was bundled into my portmanteau, without the purification of air or water, and I was obliged to depart in the dirty shirt which I had now worn for a fortnight.'[72]

This purification process at release was equally a feature of the cholera era. When Mark Twain testified to the choking nausea of fumigation in northern Italy in the 1860s, he might not have been aware it had been going on for decades. In 1832, Nathaniel Willis eagerly awaited his release from Villa Franca and was dismayed at the sight of the physician preparing an iron pot in the middle of the room and then closing the windows.

> 'The *chlorine* soon filled the room, and its detestable odour became so intolerable that we forced the door and rushed past the sentinel into the open air, nearly suffocated. This farce over, we were suffered to embark, and, rounding the point, put into Nice.'[73]

Once out of the lazaretto, travellers were normally free to do as they wished, but there could be complications. At Constantinople it was polite 'to pay a visit of ceremony to the Bey or Governor of the quarantine establishment'.[74] This passed off in a haze of pipe smoke and a slurp of coffee, and similar social events were not unknown at other quarantine stations on the borders of the Ottoman Empire. At Rothenturn, the director of the lazaretto allowed the Comte de Lagarde two days' remission on his quarantine coupled with an invitation to dinner on the day of his release.[75] On Malta, the best-connected detainees might expect to dine with the governor once their quarantine had ended, but in most western ports the authorities were only too pleased to send travellers on their way.

For some people, however, the formalities were still not over, especially at the borders of Austria. Customs regulations could be niggling both before quarantine and after. Certain items, for instance cigars at Trieste, were liable to duty on arrival and officials had an excuse to be deeply inquisitive. At Semlin and Orsova, those who left the rigid discipline of the lazaretto went straight into a troublesome follow-up. 'The custom-house at Semlin', warned John Murray, 'is particularly annoying, and every officer not only expects, but enforces a bribe'.[76] Francis Hervé had a bad experience there, not so much from the venality of officials as from their ignorance. When he left the lazaretto, he was told that his several hundred miniatures and drawings had to be sent to Vienna for inspection. He escaped paying duty on them as he was not staying in the country, but was charged three halfpence per item for carriage, which he later learnt was improper.[77] He never got his money back.

At Orsova, Captain Best found that a dollar to the clerk of the customs house 'got over every difficulty' of examining the baggage once it had left the lazaretto.[78] His books, however, had to be packed in sealed boxes and sent on to Vienna, like the artwork of Francis Hervé. Best was sardonic: 'The Austrian government, in its paternal regard for the welfare of its subjects, carefully examines every book before it is allowed to be read'.[79] When the traveller entered Austria from Moldavia, the customs service had the power, unusually, to fumigate baggage in the absence of a regular lazaretto. Edmund Spencer found the process 'calculated to make a deep inroad into the purse of any traveller . . . as every article, however small, is charged separately a kreutzer, nearly a halfpenny'.[80] According to the rules, Spencer should have surrendered his firearms at the frontier, as he had no special permission to take them through Austria, but the customs officer overlooked this infringement.

For the manuscript of his book, however, which he called 'the fruits of my industry at the quarantine of Galatz', Spencer had a torrid time. The customs officer was not prepared to let it through as it might be 'revolutionary or dangerous to the Austrian empire'. The text was, therefore, sent by special messenger for inspection by the governor of Czernowitz. 'Like Noah's dove', wrote Spencer,

> 'the ill-starred MS. found no rest; for, being written in short-hand, and intermingled with Turkish, Tartar, and Circassian words, neither the

> governor nor the whole of the learned professors of that town could decipher a single word; it was therefore sealed, and transmitted to a higher tribunal, for the perusal of the governor-general of Galicia, at Lemberg.'

Eventually, Spencer was told that the text was lost, which he took to mean it was suppressed because nobody could understand it and their suspicions remained. Luckily for him, he had sent most of his papers to England by sea from Constantinople, so the loss was not a disaster.[81]

Another vexed traveller was the Revd Justin Perkins, entering Russian territory from Turkey in 1834. He had offended the local customs officer by asking, when in quarantine, if the latter could call immediately to make the necessary examination of his books, as their packing cases had already been opened (in fact broken to bits) for the purpose of fumigation. The reply came that the man was too busy, but this was later revealed as an excuse. When the day came for pratique, the local governor asked the customs officer to expedite the examination of effects, so that Perkins and his wife could continue their journey with minimal delay. But this upset the customs officer even more, and he deliberately took his time and raised difficulties, insisting on a list of the clergyman's books. As a title such as 'Poole's *Synopsis*' meant nothing to him, he wanted the list translated into Russian, which no one could do. In the end, the man became as tired as Perkins of the pettiness of the scrutiny and let them through. Perkins was phlegmatic about the delay and attributed the 'very malevolent disposition' of the customs officer to 'his ardent devotion at the shrine of Bacchus'.[82]

Despite the evidence of some degree of contentment, most travellers found the quarantine experience irksome to say the least and wished it good riddance. Eliot Warburton welcomed 'the elasticity of restored freedom' as he stepped out from his 'imprisonment' at the Beirut lazaretto.[83] Edward Montague thought his detention at Port Mahon had been 'enough to try the patience of Job himself'.[84] Others were just bewildered and depressed after a confinement longer and harsher than they had ever imagined. George Ticknor described those departing from quarantine at Castel Franco, competing for space in a carriage, as 'like the poor souls in Virgil who are not permitted to pass over the Styx'.[85]

For others, the release from quarantine was more a cause for positive celebration than a feeling of quiet relief. Captain Frankland, returning from Russia in 1831, had found himself quarantined with others on a steamer in the harbour of Carlscrona, Sweden, during the second cholera pandemic. When news of imminent release was spread abroad, the occasion would not pass unnoticed:[86]

> 'The passengers are all wild with joy. In the evening we dressed up a figure to represent the Quarantine, and buried it with mock *Miserere* and *De profundis*; the passengers mostly dressed in white sheets, holding tapers,

> preceded by a high priest and his deacon, chanting, and sprinkling the figure with lustral water. The Devil rose through the quarter-deck skylight, and claimed the defunct as his legitimate prey. Afterwards, a ball and supper, to terminate the evening, was given by Neptune, Vulcan, and Mercury. We swam in champagne, punch, &c.'

In the morning, the port surgeon came alongside asking who was the person whose decease had been the subject of such rites and of what disorder had he died? Luckily, he found the explanation rather funny, but port officials attached to the quarantine service were not noted for their sense of humour. In fact, joviality was in short supply all round. It was not as if most people believed there was any point in the system. For the British, in particular, it went against the grain. Quarantine seemed alien to national values. Merchants felt it jarred with freedom of trade and travellers with the freedom of the individual. When applied at home, it seemed imposed only to conform with continental practice and keep British ships in free pratique abroad. With that mindset, travellers were in no mood to suffer a punitive and expensive affront to civil liberty, especially when the medical rationale seemed increasingly flimsy. For most it was an excruciating ordeal and a demeaning waste of time.

In the modern resurgence of quarantine, what has changed? Is it the same arbitrary, unsettling and negative experience which it used to be? Yes, it can hardly be otherwise, although the comparison with literal imprisonment would now be unkind, and widespread vaccination is making it less likely. What has changed most is the perception of the point of greatest risk. This was traditionally ascribed to merchandise rather than people, with the unfortunate result that in some quarters the protection of trade seemed a greater priority than public health. During the eighteenth century, for example, there was a significant demand in the West for textiles from places in the Near East where bubonic plague was endemic; in Britain there was also a strong demand for naval stores from the Baltic where plague was sporadic. Any interruption to trade from either source brought anguished howls from the City of London, chartered companies, shipowners, shipbrokers, the Navy Board and others with some vested interest.

People, most evidently, were also vectors of disease, but the number arriving from the Near East or the Baltic who were not crew or military was relatively low. For this reason, most quarantine establishments in the West were punctiliously equipped for the depuration of cargoes and catered for people only as an ancillary and unwelcome complication. Britain was more than happy for its citizens – and sometimes the cargoes of its ships – to be detained or purified in the Mediterranean lazarettos at the whim of the local administration.

In the nineteenth century, with the onset of universal cholera (and to a lesser extent yellow fever, imported in fast steamers from the Americas and West Indies), there was a change in attitude. Little or no risk was perceived from merchandise, and the quarantine of cargoes was all but eliminated except – furthering the doctrine of contagion – when there was a threat of bubonic plague. The focus was now on the health of the populace by improvements in sanitation and the removal of squalor. It was as well that cholera arrived when the mood for municipal reform was at its strongest. People were now the focus of concern, and the western world, especially Britain, gave them its full attention while commercial cargoes went on their way with little impediment.

But in another sense, the individual was the loser as government (the Privy Council being largely sidelined) was only interested in the wider picture. It was little different on the continent, which lagged behind the reforming zeal in Britain. The measures introduced were to protect the populace as an unembodied whole. Diseased vessels with horribly sick persons could still be harried from one port to another with no permission to land the dead or dying, a situation no better than it had been in earlier centuries when a ship might be fired upon to keep it out of port. The individual was expendable for the greater safety of the many. Diseases were treated by broad and brutal exclusion, and the traveller played a Russian roulette of being in the wrong vessel at the wrong time. By the later nineteenth century, a system of onboard medical inspection had done away with the worst of the horrors, and the sick were at last landed and taken to hospital.

The Covid-19 pandemic has produced two echoes of the past. The first is a vindication of contagionism, in that fear of transmission by casual touch (say, by opening a door or handling a package) seems to have advanced little from the philosophy of the eighteenth century, except now it has the backing of scientific research. The second is that the overriding concern of government is still with an abstract, if laudable, aim: this time it is the ability of hospitals to cope with an unprecedented concentration of patients. The protection of a national institution can only be assured by restricting personal liberties. If that demotion, so to speak, of the individual sounds like an alarming reversion to nineteenth-century values, of course it is not. The most vulnerable in society have been identified, prioritized and protected, a logistical exercise of monumental complexity. And emerging to help keep the hospitals in control and pre-empt the ingenuity of the invisible enemy, quarantine has risen smirking from the recesses of legality where it has dozed with one eye open for a century and a half.

The unfortunate people quarantined under Covid-19 rules could have drawn comfort that their frustration is no stronger than it was for a traveller in the Mediterranean in centuries past. May their rancour be assuaged by the stinging couplet of Lord Byron:[87]

Adieu, thou damned'st quarantine,
That gave me fever, and the spleen!

Notes

See general note as to references stated at the end of Chapter 1.

1 Plaisted (1757, 150).
2 Sandys (1673, 177–8).
3 Brydone (1790, i, 50–1).
4 Morritt (1914, 244).
5 Gell (1823, 393–4).
6 Twain (1875, 340–52).
7 Klaproth (1814, 394–6).
8 Dumont (1705, 351–4).
9 Browne (1867, 308).
10 Minet (1958, 424).
11 Warburton (1845, ii, 365).
12 Vane (1844, 164).
13 Buckingham and Chandos (1862, iii, 101–4).
14 Temple (1836, i, 165–6).
15 Kinglake (1844, 2).
16 Purchas (1905, 91–2).
17 Evers (1784, 150–1).
18 Johnes (1859, 136).
19 Najaf (1839, i, 216).
20 Slade (1840, 215).
21 Ibid., 313.
22 Giraudeau (1835, 396).
23 Birmingham City Archives, Galton MSS., 3101/C/E/5/17/51.
24 Perkins (1843, 124).
25 Ros (1855, 68–9).
26 Stuart (1854, 365).
27 Turner (1820, i, 170–1).
28 Casanova (1958–60, i, 203).
29 Wittman (1803, 421).
30 Morritt (1914, 257–8).
31 Tischendorff (1847, 282).
32 Warburton (1845, ii, 388).
33 Demidoff (1855, ii, 317).
34 Forbin (1819a, 76).
35 Lushington (1829, 198).
36 Rooke (1783, 124).
37 Stuart (1854, 361).
38 Sherer (1825, 215).
39 Waring (1843, 69).
40 Auldjo (1835, 241).
41 Griffith (1845, i, 98).
42 Montefiore (1890, i, 48).
43 Turner (1820, iii, 332).
44 Usborne (1840, 33).
45 British Library, Add. MS. 36448, ii, 4 July 1840.
46 Best (1842, 322–3).
47 Tobin (1855, 141).
48 Nerval (1851, i, 314).
49 Formby (1843, 71).
50 Hervé (1837, ii, 335).

51 Murray (1840, 217–18).
52 Walsh (1829, 317–18).
53 Spencer (1838, ii, 198); Pfeiffer (1851, 266).
54 Pfeiffer (1852, 218), Monk (1851, ii, 154).
55 Murray (1840, 16).
56 Wilkinson (1847, xxiv).
57 Fane (1842, ii, 319).
58 Woburn Abbey Collection, 6th Duke, Vouchers, 4/27/5.
59 Slatter (1984, 78).
60 Plaisted (1757, 151).
61 Montefiore (1890, i, 264).
62 Pfeiffer (1852, 218).
63 Evers (1784, 154).
64 Bryant (1869, 166–7).
65 Galton (1908, 54).
66 Waring (1843, 71–2).
67 Auldjo (1835, 243).
68 Best (1842, 324).
69 Jesse (1841, i, 61–2).
70 Terry (1848, 256).
71 Slade (1840, 321–2).
72 Walsh (1829, 317–18).
73 Willis (1850, 14).
74 Fisk (1844, 420).
75 Lagarde (1824, 361).
76 Murray (1840, 218).
77 Hervé (1837, ii, 333).
78 Best (1842, 324).
79 Ibid., 325.
80 Spencer (1838, ii, 261).
81 Ibid., 262–3.
82 Perkins (1843, 124–6).
83 Warburton (1845, ii, 64).
84 Montague (1849, 90).
85 Ticknor (1876, ii, 47).
86 Frankland (1832, ii, 458).
87 Byron (1855, ii, 318).

Gazetteer

Quarantine stations and lazarettos

This is an alphabetical gazetteer of the main places in Europe and nearby where quarantine for travellers was conducted, based on the works cited in the bibliography. It does not include (a) quarantine stations conceived specifically to beat cholera, as they were virtually universal in the nineteenth-century pandemics; (b) minor checkpoints (e.g. Taganrok on the Sea of Azov) without proper facilities; or (c) quarantine ports for military use (e.g. Toulon).

The dates refer to the period of the traveller's experience and not to the year of publication of his or her book. In the references, however, the date of publication is given to marry with the bibliography.

QS means Quarantine Station, and the number refers to the author's maps.

DOI: 10.4324/9781003195733-7

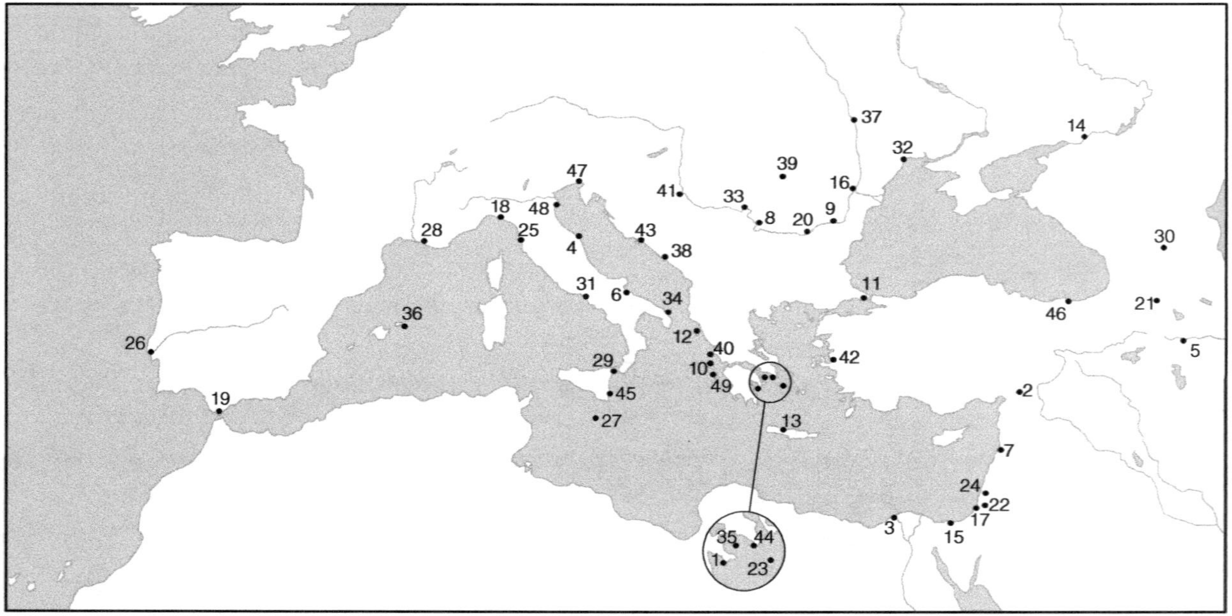

1. Aegina
2. Aintab
3. Alexandria
4. Ancona
5. Aras, River
6. Barletta
7. Beirut
8. Calafat
9. Calorash
10. Cephalonia
11. Constantinople
12. Corfu
13. Crete
14. Earlik
15. El Arish
16. Galatz
17. Gaza
18. Genoa
19. Gibraltar
20. Giurgevo
21. Gumry
22. Hebron
23. Hydra
24. Jerusalem
25. Leghorn
26. Lisbon
27. Malta
28. Marseilles
29. Messina
30. Mozdok
31. Naples
32. Odessa
33. Orsova, Old
34. Otranto
35. Piraeus
36. Port Mahon
37. Pruth, River
38. Ragusa
39. Rothenthurn
40. Santa Maura
41. Semlin
42. Smyrna
43. Spalatro
44. Syra
45. Syracuse
46. Trebizond
47. Trieste
48. Venice
49. Zante

Map 1 Major quarantine stations of the Mediterranean Basin and beyond. For details of each station, with travellers' comments, see the alphabetical list to follow.

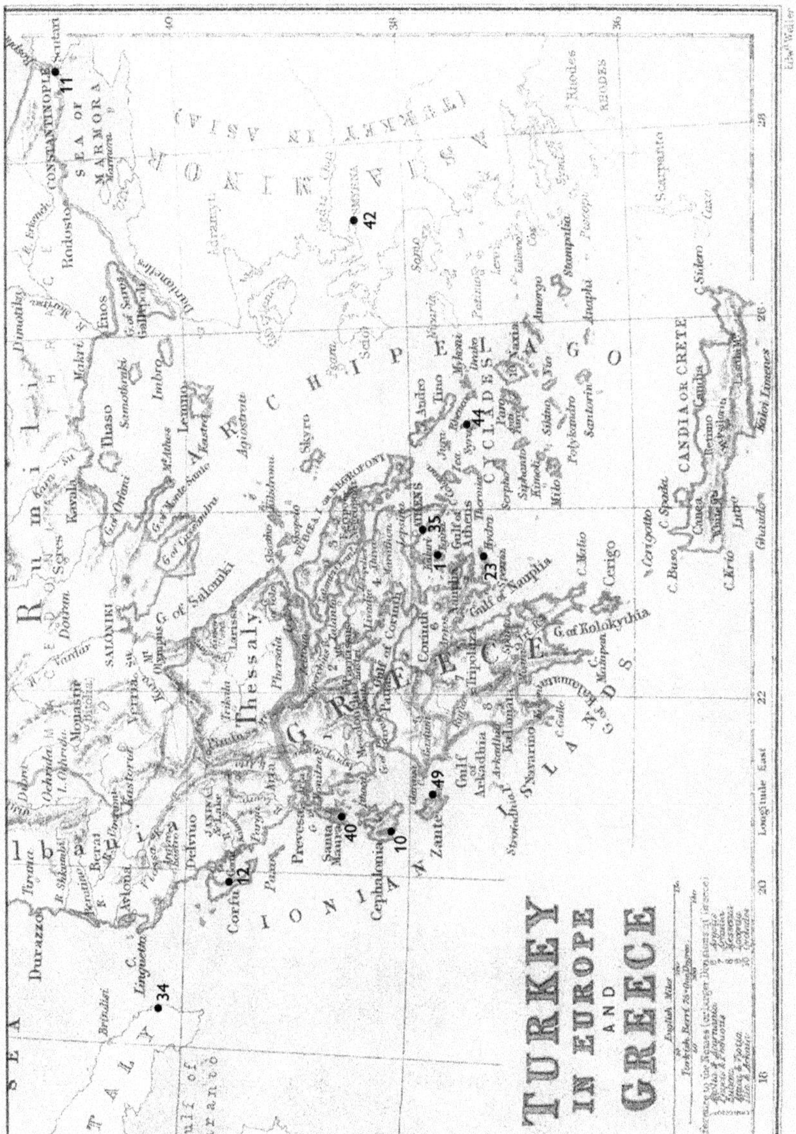

Map 2 Quarantine stations in and near Greece shown in greater details, imposed on a map of c. 1870.

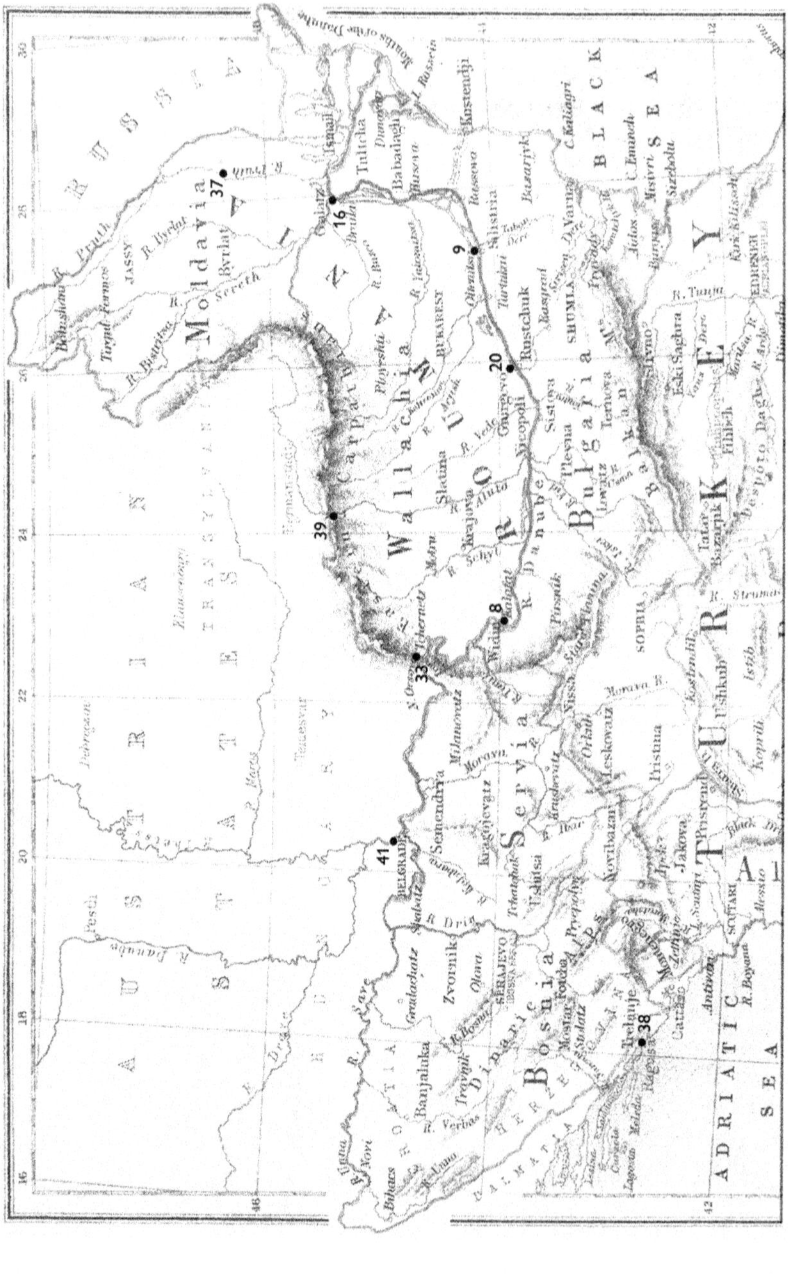

Map 3 Quarantine stations along, and near, the Danube Basin, imposed on a map of c. 1870.

AEGINA

QS number: 1

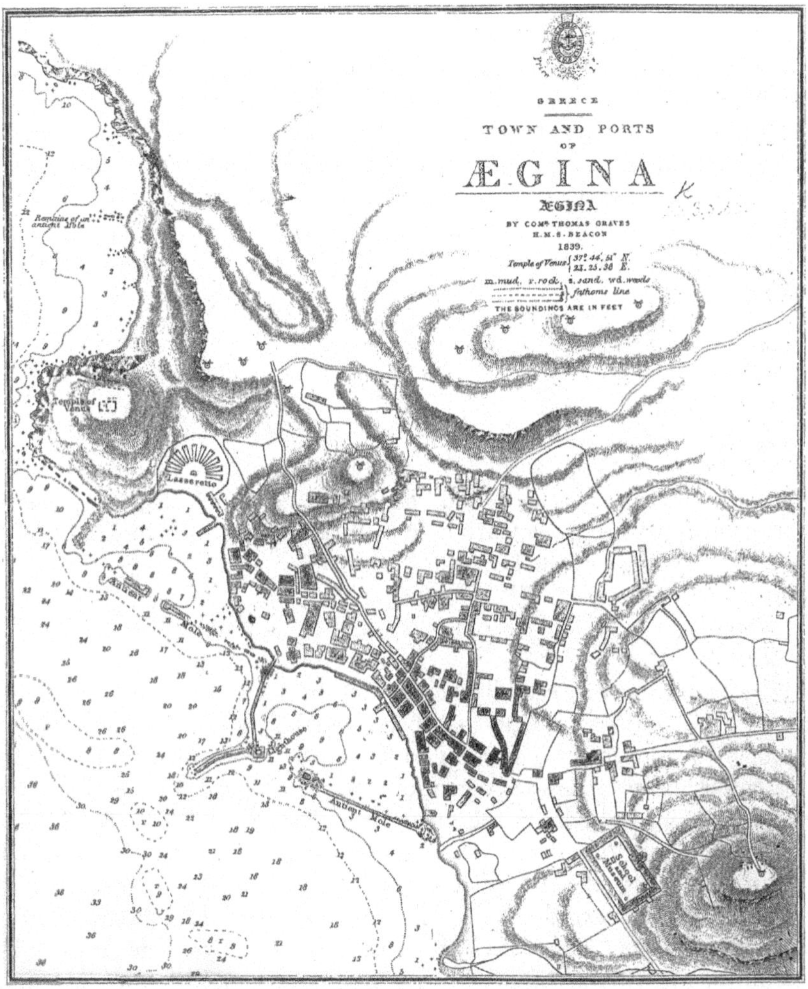

Illustration 1 Map of Aegina showing the location and layout of the fan-shaped lazaretto.

Source: © The British Library Board, Maps SEC.5.(1514)

Controlling state: Greece
Situation: Island in the Saronic Gulf, 17 miles from Athens
Sources: Trant (1829), Murray (1840), Pfeiffer (1848)

Comments:

This was conceived as the quarantine station for Athens before a lazaretto was built at Piraeus. Trant found that the facilities were recent and that quarantine was nominal.[1] Murray labelled the lazaretto as 'good', containing 'some tolerable rooms', although provisions came from Piraeus which was, in any case, set to supersede it.[2] Pfeiffer, however, found the lazaretto still open but was distinctly unimpressed by her tiny, unlit cage and the cramped space for exercise. She resented the charges for every conceivable service.[3]

AINTAB

QS number: 2

Controlling state: Syria (within Ottoman Empire)
Situation: Quarantine was initially in the village of Tel-Bascher, about 12 miles from Aintab (now Gaziantep in Turkey), at the crossing of the river Sajur, a tributary of the Euphrates.
Sources: Poujoulat (1837), Walpole (c. 1850)

Comments:

The quarantine was established by Mehemet Ali at the extreme north-east of Syria on the strategic road between Aleppo and Mosul. Poujoulat approached from the east in a state of exhaustion and was appalled to find no facilities for his seven-day detention: '*Pas une seule cabane ne se rencontre*', so he slept virtually in the open air under a ripped tent. For food he had nothing but '*du mauvais pain noir et quelques grappes de raisin*'. His pleas for lodging in the village were initially turned down, so he enlisted the support of a European doctor at Aintab, who achieved the desired accommodation, but only with difficulty, for the last four days of detention.[4] The quarantine for Walpole was also near the river Sajur but virtually in Aintab: 'We occupied one large room, windy and ruinous, but retaining many marks of former splendour; faded arabesques, gilded scrolls, and a handsome fire-place – for this was formerly the Governor's palace, and this his favourite room'. Walpole also pitched a tent on the terrace of a neighbouring khan (inn), which 'formed a quiet room to retire to, and its cool shade was peculiarly grateful'.[5]

ALEXANDRIA

QS number: 3

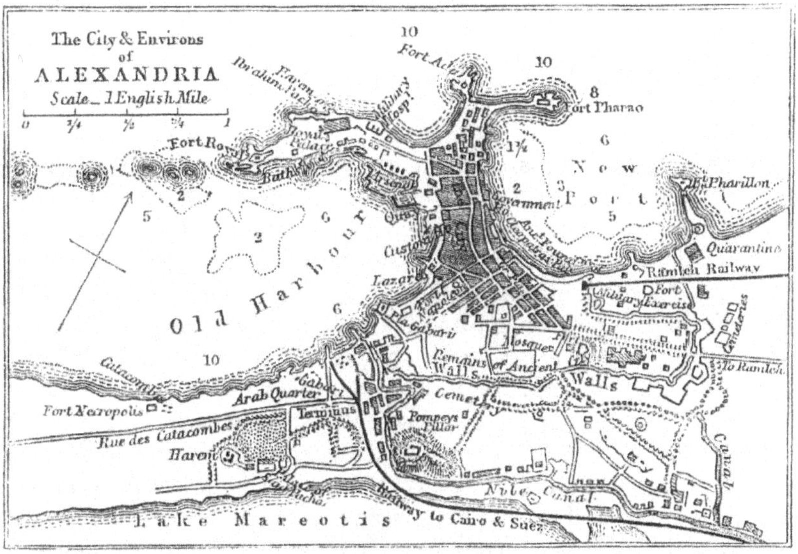

Illustration 2 Port of Alexandria c. 1870. The old 'Lazaret' is shown on the eastern side of the Old Harbour, while the newer quarantine station is marked to the east of the New Port.

Source: *Imperial Gazetteer* (London, Glasgow & Edinburgh, 1878)

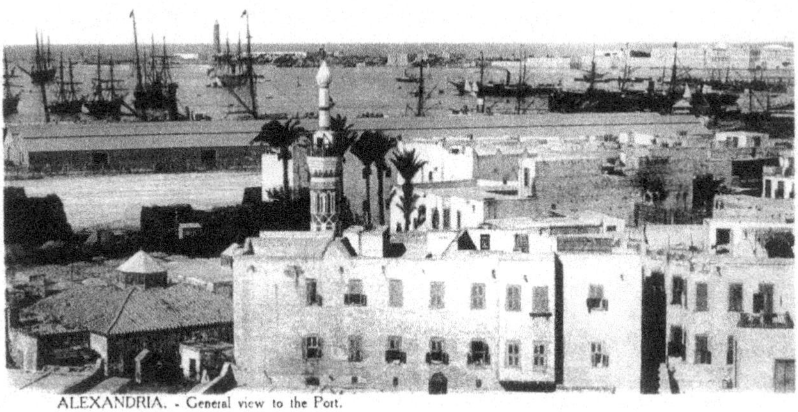

Illustration 3 The Old Harbour at Alexandria in around 1900. The original lazaretto was a little to the right of the picture on the water's edge.

Source: postcard

Controlling state: Egypt (within Ottoman Empire)
Situation: Mediterranean seaport
Sources: Wittman (1802), Bramsen (1814), Sherer (1822), D'Estourmel (1833), Macbrair (1834), Scott (1834), Marmont (1834), Bowring (1838), Robinson (1838), Pfeiffer (1842), Warburton (1843), Carlisle (1853), Beamont (1854), Maxwell (1881)

Comments:

Wittman camped in quarantine tents 'without the walls of the lazaretto', but Bramsen found all quarantine had been abolished by order of the Porte, so that Sherer performed a non-mandatory quarantine in the house of the British consul while awaiting passage to Malta.[6] In fact, there was no proper lazaretto at Alexandria until 1829 (Scott). D'Estourmel mentioned a '*lazaret*' at Alexandria with an extraordinary 91 days' quarantine against England '*parce que dans le Levant on compte plus avec le choléra qu'avec la peste*'.[7] Macbrair passed a 'very damp and uncomfortable' week of quarantine in a 'castle . . . situated in the sea' despite undergoing the *spoglio*.[8] Scott explained that the lazaretto was 'situated on the shore of the eastern harbour, outside the walls of the city'.[9] Marmont, in deference to his social standing, was allowed to pass his quarantine in a palace by the sea, owned by the Pasha.[10] That presumably went down badly with the European consuls who, as Bowring explained, controlled quarantine at Alexandria.[11]

Despite this involvement of their fellow countrymen, westerners (e.g. Warburton and Carlisle) were generally scornful of Egyptian policy, which seemed to embarrass other Levantine states deliberately. They were also distrustful of conditions. Robinson 'preferred to remain on board, rather than venture the discomforts and risks of an Egyptian lazaretto'.[12] Ida Pfeiffer 'had expected to find neither comfort nor pleasure in the quarantine-house' and was correct on both counts.[13] Her room was completely unfurnished, but at least it was cheap and the lazaretto was kept clean and tidy. Beamont was dismayed by the story of someone who, in the course of quarantine at Alexandria, was nearly drowned in the transfer from ship to shore, only 'to be afterwards nearly famished in the Lazaretto'.[14] Yachtsman Maxwell and his shipmates were ordered to the lazaretto but refused to go, remaining stubbornly 'among our own possessions in our comfortable floating home'.[15]

ANCONA
QS number: 4

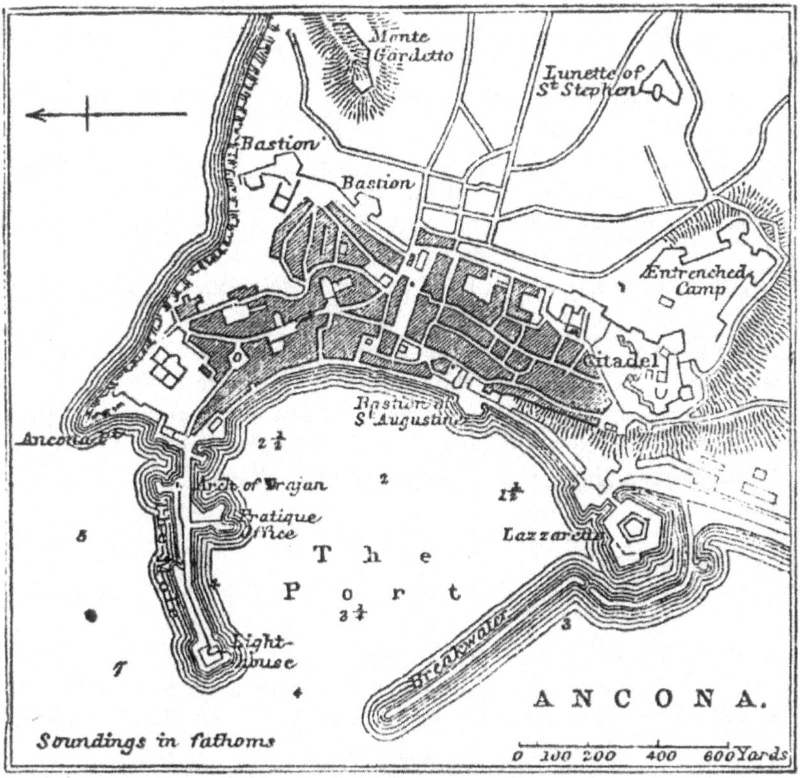

Illustration 4 Port of Ancona c. 1870. The lazaretto is indicated to the south of the harbour.

Source: *Imperial Gazetteer* (London, Glasgow & Edinburgh, 1878)

Controlling state: Papal States (but France 1832–8)
Situation: Italian Adriatic seaport
Sources: Casanova (1744), Olivier (1798), Alcock (1829), Mure (1838), Scharf (1840), Pridham (1849), Panzac (1986)

Comments:

One of the historic quarantine ports of Europe. The first two lazarettos were sixteenth century, followed by a third from the seventeenth.[16] The fourth lazaretto was purpose built to designs by the architect Luigi Vanvitelli, commissioned by Pope Clement XII and completed in 1743. Set on the edge of the sea so as to form a small island, the pentagonal building was surrounded by a walkway and a high perimeter wall, resembling both a barracks and a prison. The romantic machinations of Casanova took place in the third lazaretto, which continued in use until 1748. Despite these buildings, brief quarantines could evidently be passed on board ship in the late eighteenth century.[17] Quarantine was maintained against arrivals from the Levant via the Ionian Islands despite stringent detentions at Corfu, simply to appease French and Austrian demands.[18] The lazaretto could be almost deserted in the late 1830s:

> 'The whole establishment being at our disposal, we enjoyed all the freedom and comfort compatible with its limits and regulations. We had each as much house-room as we cared to occupy. Our meals were served at reasonable rates from the best hotel in the town.'[19]

Scharf called the lazaretto 'a good square isolated building protected by a drawbridge',[20] while Pridham thought it among the few 'fine edifices and public works' in a town which in other respects was 'about the truest picture of squalor and brutality the human eye could light upon'.[21] The lazaretto was disused from about 1860 but the building still exists.

ARAS, RIVER

QS number: 5

Controlling state: Russia
Situation: The boundary between Persia and Russia, north of Tabriz, now the boundary between Iran and Azerbaijan
Sources: Macintosh (1837), Wilbraham (1837)

Comments:

Macintosh crossed by ferry to the quarantine station, 'a group of ten or twelve miserable mud-huts, dug on the side of the bank'.[22] He was allowed out to visit the historic ruins of nearby Julfa. Wilbraham crossed the Aras at much the same time:

> 'I looked in vain for the building of the quarantine establishment, the only house visible being a small square hut, the residence of the superintendent. On landing I found that the sole accommodation for travellers consisted in some half-dozen subterranean cells, low and dark, and swarming with cockroaches. I was ushered into one of these, which had been carpeted with red baize, and contained the luxuries of a table and chair, though of the most primitive and least comfortable construction.'[23]

Both Macintosh and Wilbraham got on well with the quarantine director.

BARLETTA

QS number: 6

Controlling state: Naples
Situation: Italian Adriatic seaport
Sources: Morritt (1795), Hughes (1813), Laurent (1819), Grellet (1819), Kinglake (1835)

Comments:

The port was linked administratively to Otranto (q.v.) and Brindisi, serving as the main quarantine centre for both. Morritt described the lazaretto as 'tolerable'.[24] Hughes found standards slack but 'had no reason . . . to complain of any want of civility in the officers of the lazaretto or in the inhabitants of the town', who brought gifts of fruit and wine.[25] Laurent found the lazaretto 'a miserable stone building, erected on a small island at one extremity of the town, to which it is united by a narrow bridge'.[26] Grellet and an English merchant were placed 'in the same apartments . . . though in a separate chamber', a considerable concession as the lazaretto was overcrowded.[27] Kinglake had the favour of a reduced detention.[28]

BEIRUT

QS number: 7

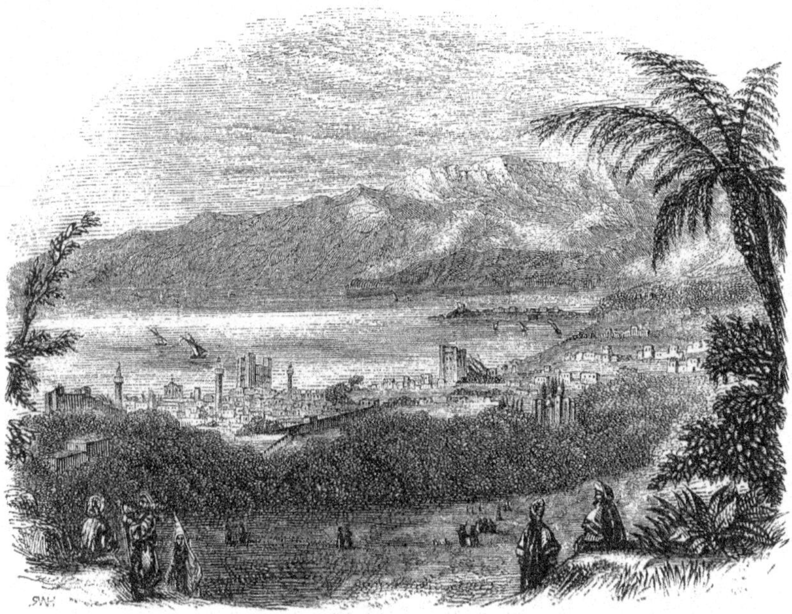

Beyroot from the South.

Illustration 5 View of Beirut. The peninsula in the middle background was the site of the lazaretto.

Source: Kelly, W., *Syria and the Holy Land* (London, 1844)

Controlling state: Syria (within Ottoman Empire)
Situation: Mediterranean seaport, now capital of Lebanon
Sources: Bowring (1838), Holroyd (1839), Millard (1842), Bowring (1842), Warburton (1843), de Nerval (1843), Kelly (1844), Galton (1845), Taylor (1852), Johnes (1859)

Comments:

Quarantine was established in the 1830s as a reciprocal inconvenience for delays at Alexandria. Any hope that this political dogfight would disappear was spoilt by the British consul, in 1840, who engineered that quarantine should continue 'simply and solely to prevent the French from communicating with the Syrian coast'.[29] The lazaretto was particularly unhealthy, with detainees dying of plague and dysentery.[30] Millard, approaching from Tyre, found quarantine at Beirut against land arrivals but not against local shipping.[31] Warburton was allowed to pass 12 days of quarantine in a three-bedroomed cottage, 'a reprieve from that great pest-house, the lazaretto, whose melancholy inmates we could see wandering to and fro upon their narrow rock'.[32] This rock, as Gérard de Nerval explained, was a peninsula: the buildings nearest the land were for airing goods, while at the extremity, directly overlooking the sea, was the lazaretto for passengers. Despite serious overcrowding and night-time mosquitoes, the weather and scenery were delightful and de Nerval found the quarantine '*fort supportable*'.[33] Kelly wondered whether the 'perfectly ineffective' quarantine was still in force.[34] Galton was quarantined with his two pet monkeys and enjoyed special privileges (including 'a champagne picnic' at sea), because the director was overawed by his 'social importance'.[35] Taylor described the site as on a headland and noted 'several rows of one-story houses overlooking the sea, each containing two empty rooms', with a more expensive 'square two-story dwelling' standing apart.[36] The barrier against the town was 'a double screen of wire, with an interval between, so that contact is impossible'.[37] Despite the lack of privacy and amenities, and a nasty fumigation, Taylor was enchanted by the setting. The comments of Johnes are so similar to those of Taylor that he was evidently a plagiarist.

CALAFAT

QS number: 8

Controlling state: Russia (nominally Wallachia)
Situation: Danube town, left bank, now in Romania
Sources: Andersen (1841), Skene (1850)

Comments:

The site was directly opposite the Turkish city of Widin (now Vidin in Bulgaria), where Andersen was 'smoked through' in 'a little wooden house' before he could enter the town.[38] The main quarantine restrictions, however, were at Calafat, where Skene crossed the Danube from Widin. He and a friend were

> 'received by the Director of the Quarantine establishment, and consigned to a room in the Lazaretto for four days; but we could not even enter this little prison without undergoing the barbarous process of the *spoglio*, which consists in leaving the suspected wardrobe in the hands of the gaolers to be aired, while other more innocent clothing is provided by them.'[39]

The director revealed to Skene that the unspoken purpose of the quarantine was to interrogate travellers and intercept mail.

CALORASH

QS number: 9

Controlling state: Russia (nominally Wallachia)
Situation: Danube village, left bank, now in Romania
Sources: Burton (1836), Elliott (c.1837)

Comments:

An insignificant place, strategically sited across the Danube from the important river port of Silistra (or Silistria) formerly in Turkey and now Bulgaria. Burton found a quarantine of 21 days for those crossing north from Silistra, and the station at Calorash was difficult to reach. 'I waded above my knees through a mass of sheep's dung, filthy straw, and water, to the lazaretto, built on an eminence above the Danube . . . in a healthy enough position' with a fumigation house.[40] Burton shared an 'apartment' with a large Jewish family as western visitors were rare. His guardian was 'astonished' that Burton had not gone farther west for his quarantine, on 'another route the English take'.[41] Elliott had the unusual misfortune to be barred from landing at Silistra from a Danube steamer when the town was held for a time by the Russians, who 'established a quarantine, more political than sanitary'.[42] It was very short-lived.

CANDIA, *SEE* CRETE

CEPHALONIA

QS number: 10

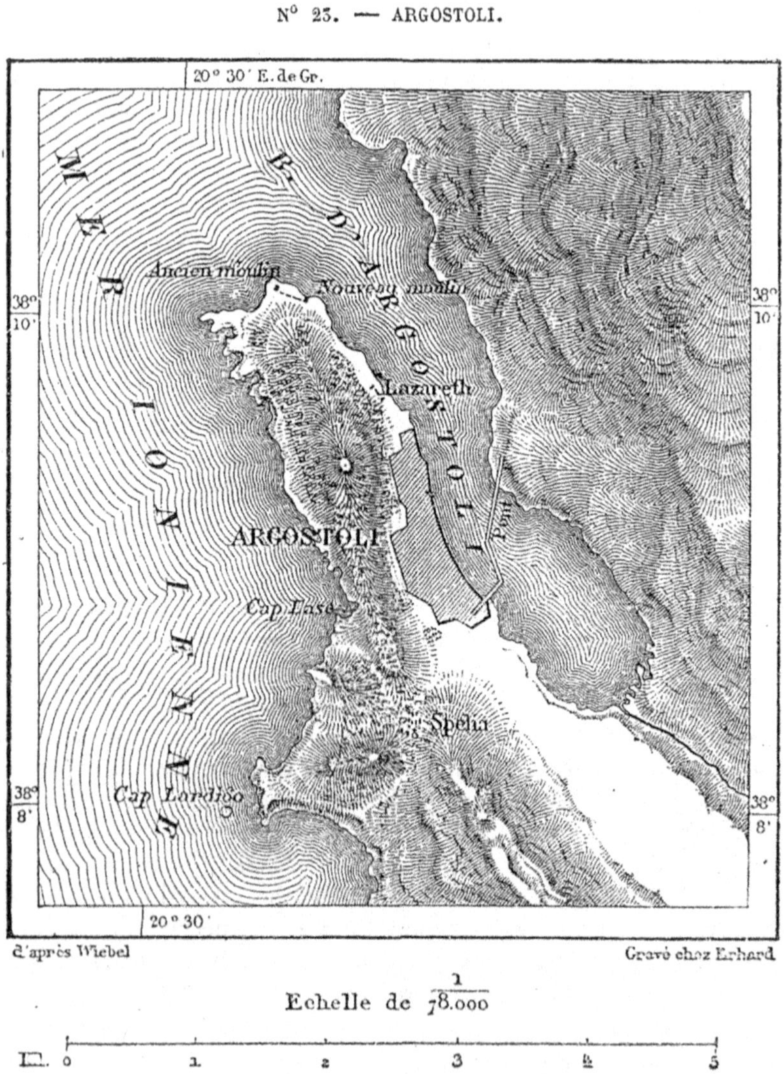

Illustration 6 Map of the Argostoli region of Cephalonia in the 1870s marking the 'Lazareth' (lazaretto) built by the British.

Source: Reclus, E., *Nouvelle Géographie Universelle* (Paris, 1876–94)

Controlling state: Venetian Republic; France from 1797; part of the Septinsular Republic from 1799; France from 1807; Britain from 1814; Greece from 1864
Situation: One of the Greek Ionian Islands, now Kefalonia
Sources: Pococke (1740), Grasset (c.1791), Panzac (1986), Booker (2007)

Comments:
The lazaretto was built at Argostoli in 1705.[43] Pococke decided to stay on his ship as he was suspicious of the facilities ashore.[44] Grasset thought the lazaretto, prominent at the harbour entrance, looked distinctly miserable ('*il n'a rien que de triste*').[45] It consisted of a small square with turrets at the corners, one side being the administration block. There was a small Greek church attached. The British built a new lazaretto in the 1820s, and the original building was demolished around 1900.[46]

CONSTANTINOPLE AND THE BOSPHORUS

QS number: 11

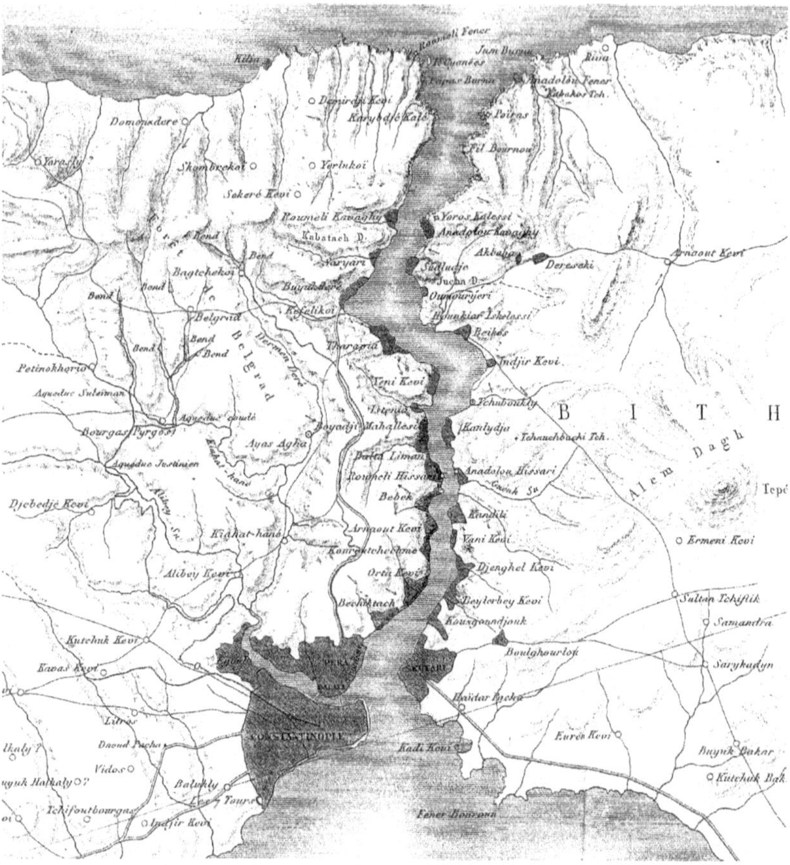

Illustration 7 Constantinople and the Bosphorus. The Golden Horn is the harbour (named after its shape) between Constantinople proper and Galata. The quarantine station of Kuleli is represented by Kandili on the map, while Kavak is shown as Anadolou Kavaghy. Kartal, where quarantine was sometimes passed in the Sea of Marmara, is a little off the map to the bottom right.

Source: Tchihatchef, P., *Le Bosphore et Constantinople* (Paris, 1866)

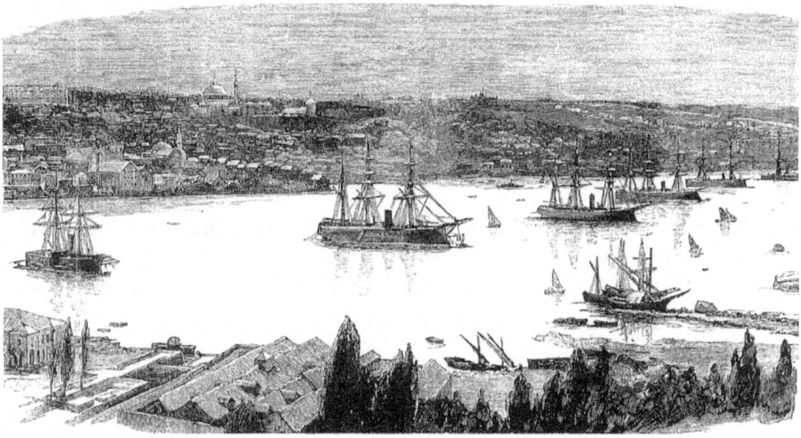

THE TURKISH FLEET IN THE "GOLDEN HORN."

Illustration 8 From the 1830s, British ships in pratique received a licence in the Golden Horn from the board of health or a consular official to proceed through the Bosphorus or Dardanelles.

Source: Spry, W., *Life on the Bosphorus* (London, 1896)

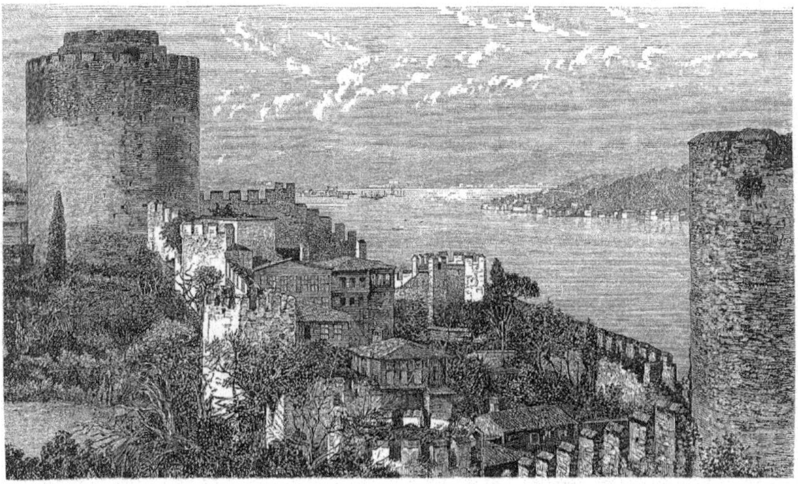

THE CASTLE OF EUROPE, ON THE BOSPHORUS.

Illustration 9 The Castle of Europe, north of Bebek on the Bosphorus, was visible from the quarantine station of Kuleli across the water.

Source: Spry, W., *Life on the Bosphorus* (London, 1896)

Controlling state: Turkey (Ottoman Empire)
Situation: Sea of Marmara; now called Istanbul. The Bosphorus links the Sea of Marmara with the Black Sea.
Sources: Tafur (1437), Bowring (1838), Best (1838), Slade (1838), Perkins (1841), Davy (1842), Stent (1842), Fisk (1842), Warburton (1843), Heywood (1845), Vigier (1885)

Comments:

For reasons discussed elsewhere in this study, quarantine was not formally introduced into Turkey until the nineteenth century. But Tafur, ironically, mentioned restrictions against Black Sea arrivals at a time when quarantine was still embryonic even in Venice: because

> 'no ships . . . were to enter the harbour . . . they built a shelter two leagues from Constantinople where the ships could discharge their cargo, and where they had to remain for sixty days unless they were prepared to put to sea again.'[47]

In the 1830s, with advice from Maltese experts and prompted by the British Government, Turkey began plans for a grand quarantine station along European lines. This never quite materialized, but many minor stations appeared along the Dardanelles and the Bosphorus over the next 20 years, none of which received a good word from physicians and politicians in the West. Bowring feared venality would be a greater spur than public health, and Best alleged that health officers 'did not exactly comprehend' that they were 'just as likely to catch or communicate plague as any one else'.[48] Slade thought the system too haphazard to be effective.[49] Perkins, on the other hand, was won over. He described his lazaretto as 'spacious, convenient and imposing', even though it had been built as barracks.[50] The site was 'five or six miles above the harbor on the Asiatic shore of the Bosphorus', which identifies it as the lazaretto of Kuleli, one of several within a few hours of the city. Davy visited there at much the same time, where he was startled to see a doctor dressing a suppurating bubo with his bare fingers and then taking a pinch of snuff 'without even washing his hands'.[51]

Stent was also at Kuleli. He was unimpressed by the ramshackle furniture and the fleas, but the buildings were 'delightfully situated' with a fine view.[52] Fisk was possibly in the same establishment – 'a large prison-like building, as filthy as can well be imagined'.[53] He cursed the rats and the vermin and the 'loathsome' hygiene. Warburton was at the lazaretto of Kartal on the Asiatic shore of the Sea of Marmara, but he was no more enamoured of the building: 'Travellers! Avoid Kartal as you would the plague that it professes to be a guard against'.[54] He was given 'a large, empty room, with discoloured walls, and a floor thickly covered with dirt and gravel, among which ants and fleas were swarming'.[55] Heywood stated that his lazaretto was at Cavak (more normally Kavak), on the Asiatic side of the Bosphorus overlooking the Black Sea and two hours' travel from Constantinople.[56] He made frequent delightful excursions to the Genoese Castle, from which the views towards the Black Sea were breathtaking. The regime appears to have been especially lax, and only the inevitable vermin spoiled what was almost a vacation. Kavak must correspond with the fishing village of Anadoli-Kavac mentioned by Vigier as the place where, even 40 years later, the yellow flag of quarantine barred the progress of his ship.[57] It is now the tourist village of Anadolu Kavaği.

CORFU

QS number: 12

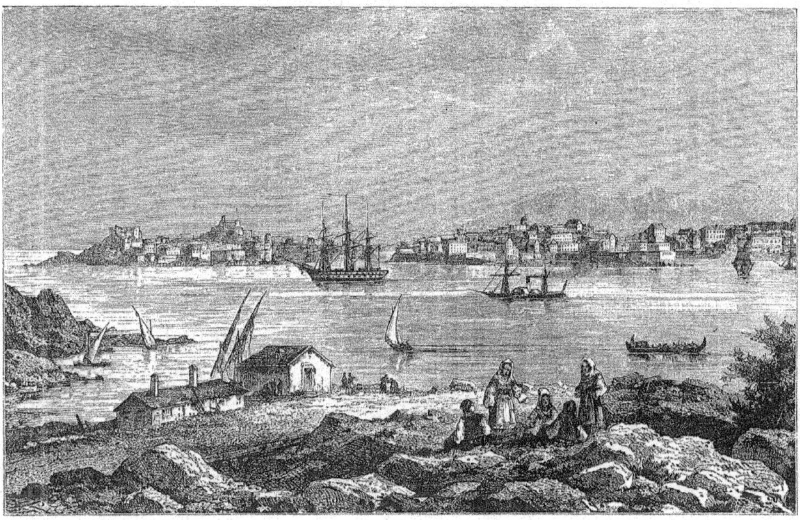

CORFU.

Illustration 10 A man-of-war and a paddle steamer in the harbour of Corfu, where quarantine was performed on an off-island.

Source: Hanson, C., *The Land of Greece Described and Illustrated* (London, 1886)

Controlling state: Venetian Republic; France from 1797; part of the Septinsular Republic from 1799; France from 1807; Britain from 1814; Greece from 1864

Situation: One of the Greek Ionian Islands, also known as Corcyra (Kerkyra)

Sources: Howard (1785), Olivier (1798), Dodwell (c.1801), Alcock (1829), Best (1838), Londonderry (1840), Lear (1849), Denison (1849), Murray (1854), Bussolin (1881), Panzac (1986)

Comments:

Howard noted that, 'The lazaretto at Corfu is finely situated on a rock surrounded with water, about a league from the city'.[58] Olivier explained that the 'rock' was one of three small islands in the bay and known as 'San-Dimitri', which Dodwell translated to 'St. Demetrius'.[59] Alcock reckoned quarantine at Corfu to be efficient, but Best discovered it could be avoided by spending the time off the Albanian coast (albeit with a health guardian) shooting at birds.[60] Lord and Lady Londonderry were allowed to stay in the health office instead of the lazaretto, 'a large, cold building on a desert island, two miles off'.[61] Both Lear and Denison found that quarantine was still imposed in 1849, but Murray placed Corfu among the four best lazarettos in the Mediterranean.[62] Bussolin, who visited the lazaretto in the late 1870s, published a ground plan showing a series of apartments on one side of a large open square, with warehouses for goods on the other side and sentry posts on two corners of the perimeter wall.[63]

CRETE

QS number: 13

Controlling state: Ottoman Empire
Situation: Eastern Mediterranean island, now part of Greece
Sources: Scott (1834)

Comments:

Under French guidance, quarantine was established in 1831 with a lazaretto at Candia (now Heraklion) in the old Venetian galley docks. Scott was conducted there with a promise that 'every attention' would be paid to his comfort.[64] He was, therefore, horrified to find 'a dark unventilated cell, on the bare walls of which rheumatism, catarrh, pleurisy, and consumption were written in ever-trickling streams of water'. Luckily he and his friend had hammocks and a tent, which they pitched within the room. They smoked and drank brandy to counteract the dampness and hired furniture from the town. But at least the view was 'splendid' and they were allowed to exercise along one of the harbour moles.

DUBROVNIK, *SEE* RAGUSA

EGARLIK
QS number: 14

Controlling state: Russia
Situation: Caucasus, at Sredne-Yegorlikskaya on the road from Stavropol to Novocherkassk
Sources: Strachey (1817), Lumsden (1820), Lyall (c. 1823)

Comments:

This was a quarantine station established for those entering the territory of the Don Cossacks from the south. Strachey had an accelerated passage through the formalities, having written to the local Cossack leader, General Count Platoff.[65] Lumsden had a similar concession from General Yermaloff, Governor of the Caucasian Provinces, and found the station 'a very handsome establishment. The only thing of which we had cause to complain was very bad water'.[66] He recalled that the lazaretto consisted of 'eleven good comfortable wooden houses, each divided into two suites of rooms, and each house separated from another by ditches and banks with good compounds; besides these, there are a great many other buildings for fumigation, &c &c'.[67] He had to 'smoke' his banknotes, apparently not to their detriment. Lyall spent three days 'at this miserable place; a title it has received from all travellers [but evidently not Lumsden], and which it well merits, notwithstanding the improvements made within the last few years'.[68] He described the situation as 'the worst imaginable, in the middle of a perfect marsh'. The near-stagnant water from the river Yegorlyk (named after 'the disagreeable odour it emits') was so bad that the quarantine physician 'sent twenty versts [about 13 miles] for all that used in his family'.[69] Lyall's description of the site was very much like Lumsden's, but he counted 'a dozen new wooden houses' and described the interiors in more detail. Each house contained 'two rooms, with a stove between them, besides an antechamber, with a large oven, which may serve as a kitchen'.[70] The quarantine station was supplied by a local merchant from whom they 'received good articles', and the regime was sufficiently lax to allow Lyall to visit the nearby village and church.[71]

EL ARISH

QS number: 15

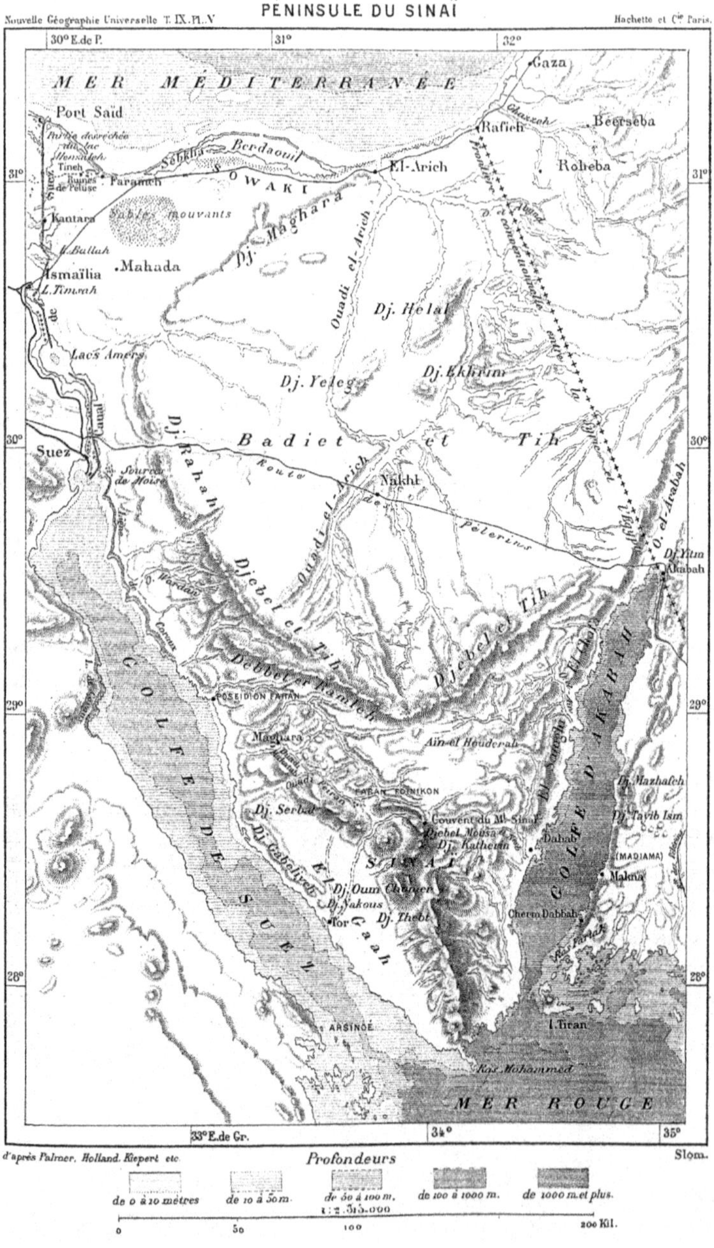

Illustration 11 With the Sinai desert being so extensive, canny travellers could bypass the quarantine at El Arish (here spelt El-Arich) by staying well to the south. The map also shows Gaza, the previous quarantine station on the journey west.

Source: Reclus, E., *Nouvelle Géographie Universelle* (Paris, 1876–94)

Controlling state: Egypt (within Ottoman Empire)
Situation: On the north coast of the Sinai peninsula
Sources: de Malherbe (1843)

Comments:

Luckily, de Malherbe struck up an immediate friendship with the Italian physician attached to the quarantine station, otherwise his detention would have been most vexing.[72] He described the lazaretto (in French) as a hideous, irregular yard surrounded by walls of dried mud, and there was no prison in Europe which would not seem a palace by comparison with that wretched slum. It was sited by a cemetery from which the sea breeze wafted nasty smells, and the only water supply came from what he described as a cesspool. He was all the more angry because (a) he came from Gaza with a certificate of good health; (b) the notion of quarantine in Egypt, '*la métropole de la peste*', was to him absurd; and (c) his guide had tricked him into arriving at the lazaretto, which might be bypassed by keeping to the south. Malherbe noted by the shore the remains of the first lazaretto, which the Egyptian ruler had intended to be large and solid, but the local work force had appropriated the bricks and built it instead of soft clay. This earlier building was knocked down by Bedouins in 1840.

GALATZ

QS number: 16

Controlling state: Russia (nominally Moldavia)
Situation: Danube river port, left bank, now in Romania
Sources: Spencer (1836), Elliott (c.1837), Best (1839), Londonderry (1840), Pfeiffer (1842), Marmier (c.1845), Carlisle (1853), Boucher de Perthes (1853)

Comments:

Best described the town as 'a good size, but its appearance from the river is not very prepossessing'.[73] The quarantine prevented him from landing for a closer inspection. Ida Pfeiffer did land but found it 'a miserable dirty place' with few women in evidence.[74] Marmier thought the town looked more like a large encampment than a centre of commerce.[75] Carlisle wondered 'not that the plague has ever got there, but that it has ever got out again'.[76] Stringent quarantine was enforced against Turkey, and the bad lazaretto was about three miles from the landing stage. Spencer endured a 'miserable cell' with a straw mattress and blanket and extortionate prices for food.[77] He found detention could be shortened by a bribe. Lord and Lady Londonderry were leaving Galatz rather than landing there but could not avoid quarantine complications in boarding the steamer.[78] Marmier found the quarantine '*un établissement sévère*', but pointless as the town was so dirty and unpaved.[79] Boucher de Perthes was pleased to have a place for his detention '*assez étendu pour un promenade*', but it lacked any view.[80] He ordered a cutlet for his lunch but received only a cup of black coffee and two biscuits.[81]

GAZA

QS number: 17

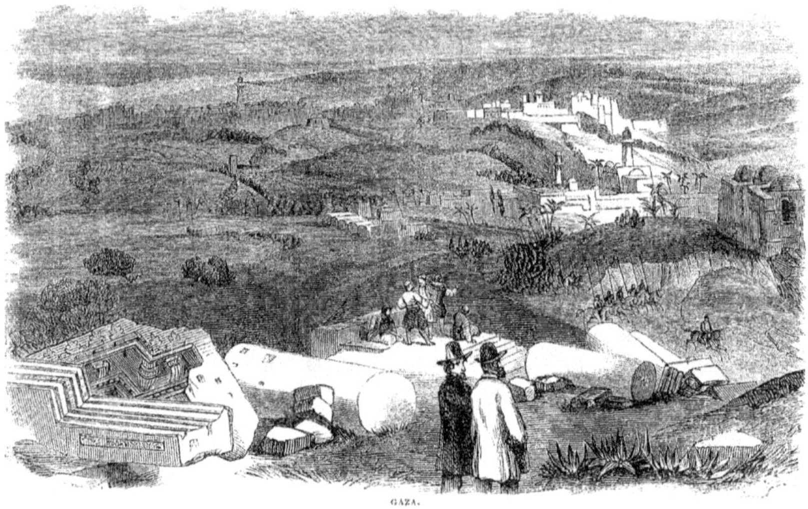

Illustration 12 Ruins at Gaza. The view gives a sense of the fragility of local stone, which was so crumbly that even the new quarantine station decayed quickly.

Source: Thomson, W., *The Land and the Book* (New York, 1859)

Controlling state: Palestine (within Ottoman Empire)
Situation: Close to Mediterranean Sea
Sources: Stent (1842), Tischendorff (1844), Spencer (1849), Neale (1850), Bryant (1853), Tobin (1854), Thomson (1857)

Comments:

Stent implied that detentions were new, justified by plague at Damietta in Egypt. He spent three days 'ruralising in the open quarantine ground pleasantly situated within a mile of Gaza'.[82] Tischendorff was annoyed to be 'quartered in miserable quarantine' after a fortnight in 'the healthy air and ventilation of the winds of the desert'.[83] His tent was pitched in old, smelly animal stalls until he persuaded the French doctor to move him. He was then 'transplanted to the roof of Ibrahim Pasha's stables', and he summed up his experience as 'the caricature of a quarantine'.[84] Spencer was detained seven days in the 'vile prison-house' of a lazaretto. 'The rooms are damp, and when it rains, wet and nasty'.[85] Neale was one of the first Franks to benefit from a large, new building, constructed under the guidance of Dr Eperon, the local French physician, as late as 1850. The lazaretto was 'in an oblong form, surrounded by walls thirty feet high. Parallel with, and some four yards separated from these walls, run the apartments allotted to strangers; the magazine for baggage, the armory, baths and incense rooms'.[86] Nearby were the offices and guard rooms, as well as 'a parlatorio, a bazaar, and a kitchen' and a very deep well. The apartments, wrote Neale, were 'so constructed as to be airy and wholesome in the summer, and warm and comfortable in winter'.[87]

Certainly Bryant had no complaints in his three-day stay. He occupied 'two small chambers' on the second floor (which existed only at each end of the building), while his attendants 'occupied a room below'.[88] Catherine Tobin was less enthusiastic during a January visit, recording that her windows had only iron bars and no glass and were closed from the outside by wooden shutters. But she was amused that the tower over the gateway was occupied by the director's harem and delighted by the quality of local fruit and vegetables. In short, her stay was not unpleasant, but she thought 'the quarantine at Gaza must be as inefficient as any other'.[89] Thomson noted an 'air of decay' over Gaza, partly because the local stone was not durable: 'On the southwest of the city are the quarantine buildings, erected by the present government out of this same description of stone, and they already show signs of decay'.[90]

GENOA

QS number: 18

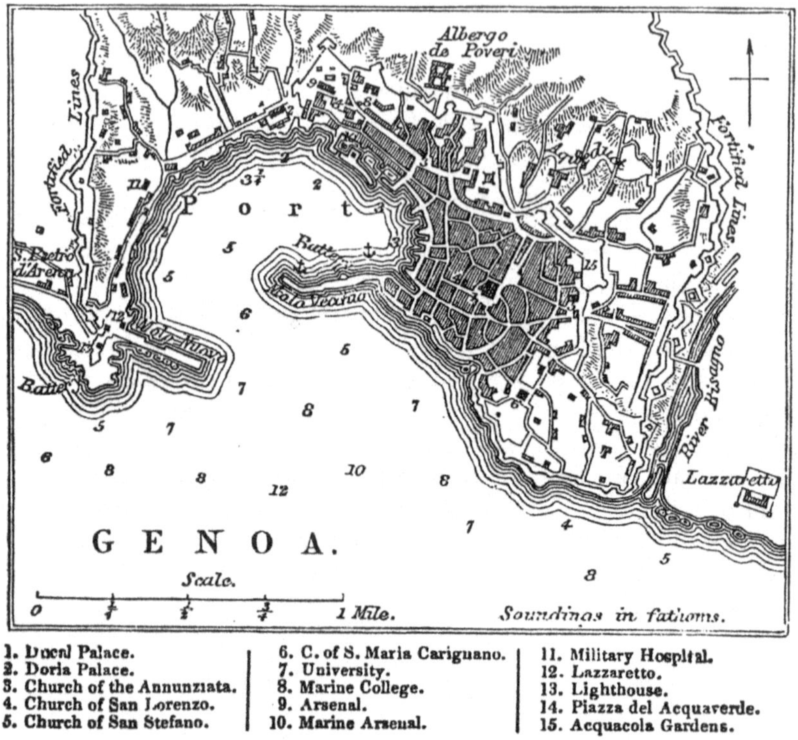

Illustration 13 Map of Genoa c. 1870. A lazaretto is shown in open country to the east of the city, while another (numbered 12) is marked to the west of the port.

Source: *Imperial Gazetteer* (London, Glasgow & Edinburgh, 1878)

Controlling state: Genoa, which existed under French protection as the Ligurian Republic from 1797; part of French Empire, 1805–14; incorporated into Kingdom of Sardinia in 1815; Kingdom of Italy, 1861
Situation: Italian Mediterranean seaport
Sources: Labat (1706), de Sainte-Maure (1721), Rousseau (1743), Howard (1785), Slade (1830), Macbrair (1833), Panzac (1986)

Comments:

Despite being a member of the select 'clique' of senior Mediterranean quarantine ports, Genoa was never much used by travellers until the age of steamers, and by then delays were minimal. Even less frequented by voyagers

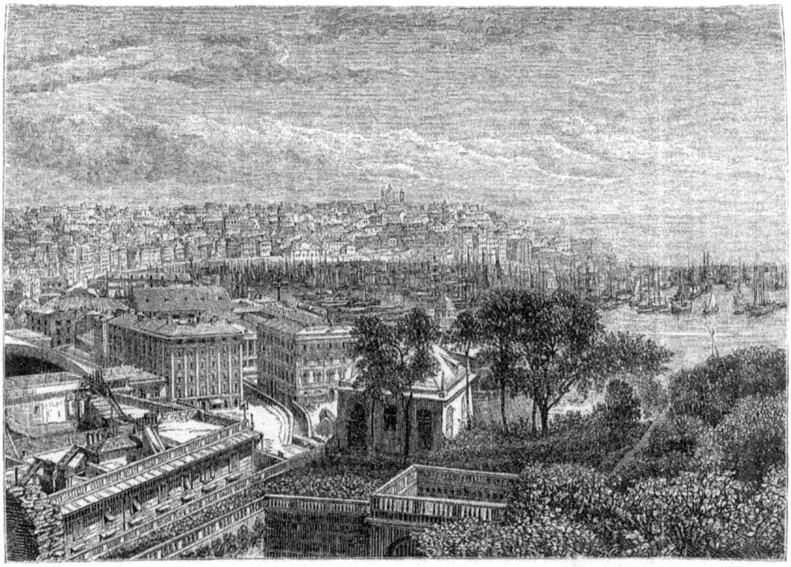
GÊNES
Dessin de J. Sorrieu, d'après une photographie de J. Lévy et Cie.

Illustration 14 Ships packed into Genoa Harbour. The health office was among the buildings in the foreground.

Source: Reclus, E., *Nouvelle Géographie Universelle* (Paris, 1876–94)

was the alternative lazaretto purpose built by the Genoese at La Spezia in the 1720s after the shock plague at Marseilles. Slade cursed the quarantine system there but did not describe the lazaretto, although moored only 'half a cable' away.[91] The site was on the peninsula of Varignano, and Panzac gives the history with plan and photographs.[92] Labat noted that quarantine services at Genoa itself were free, but because the employees were paid by the state and therefore had no perks to look forward to, they were rather surly.[93] Sainte-Maure, on the other hand, found the service expensive as well as strict, but at least his detention was brief.[94]

Rousseau, arriving from plague-stricken Messina, was given a quarantine of 21 days, later shortened to 14. Passengers on his ship were offered the choice of staying on board or disembarking for the lazaretto. Only Rousseau chose the latter course, and he literally had the place to himself. He was quartered in a large, two-storey building totally without furniture or fittings, but he made himself comfortable with his own considerable possessions. Being the sole inmate, he was at liberty to explore the building at will, and he wandered as far as the Protestant cemetery and upstairs to a lantern where he could view the harbour. At other times he amused

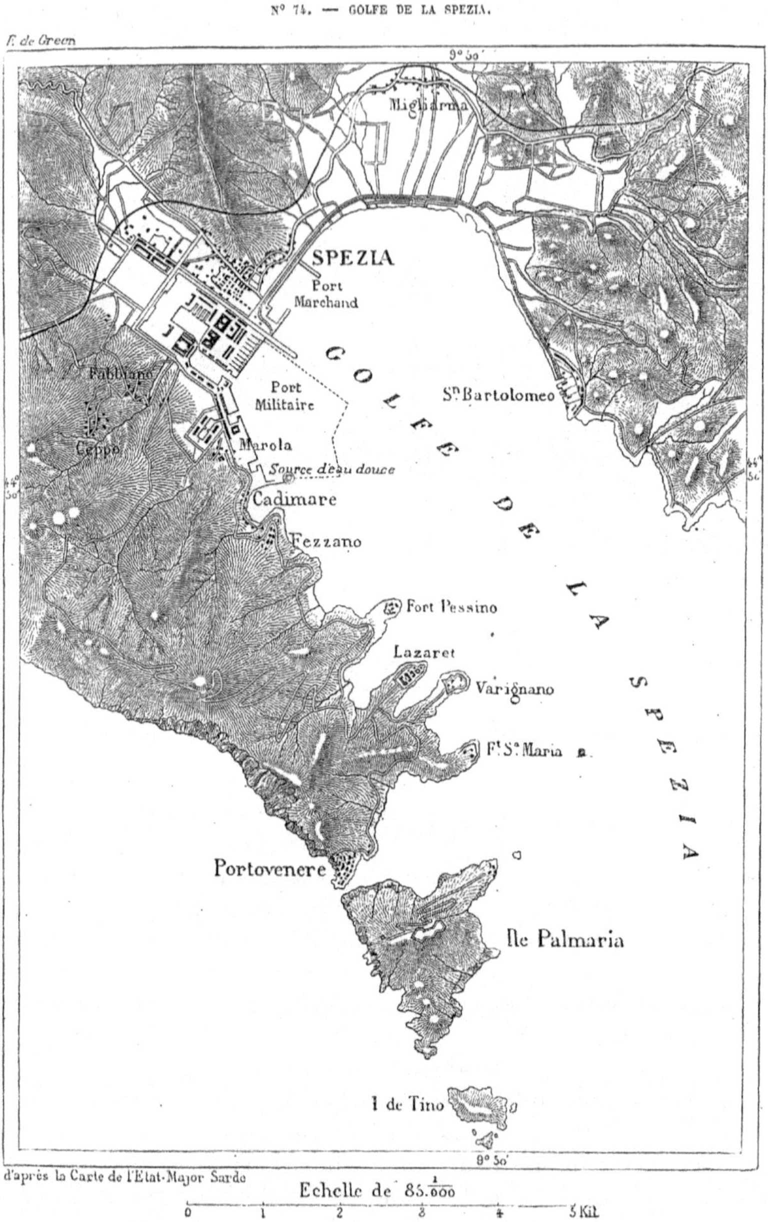

Illustration 15 The main quarantine station for Genoa was at Varignano near La Spezia. The 'Lazaret' is shown on this map from the 1870s.

Source: Reclus, E., *Nouvelle Géographie Universelle* (Paris, 1876–94)

himself by hunting fleas, as he had done on the ship, and by reading and writing. His meals were brought to him escorted by two soldiers with fixed bayonets, and he used a step for a seat and his mattress as a table. He was not at all bothered by the solitude.[95] Howard was impressed by the city lazaretto and published a view and plan. He liked the regularity of the design with a 'centre-row equally dividing the areas, which are three hundred and ten feet by twenty-five'. Most rooms were around 16 feet × 14 feet and more than 11 feet high. These rooms each had two opposite windows which had iron bars and shutters, but no glass and all were 'too small'. The floors were brick and the roofs vaulted, and each room had a chimney in one corner, and in the other 'a sewer shut in like a closet' – a very rare reference to toilet facilities.[96] Macbrair, sailing only from Marseilles, found that health and passport formalities were strict, but no attendance was necessary at the lazaretto.[97] Panzac dates demolition of the Varignano lazaretto to around 1900.[98]

GIBRALTAR

QS number: 19

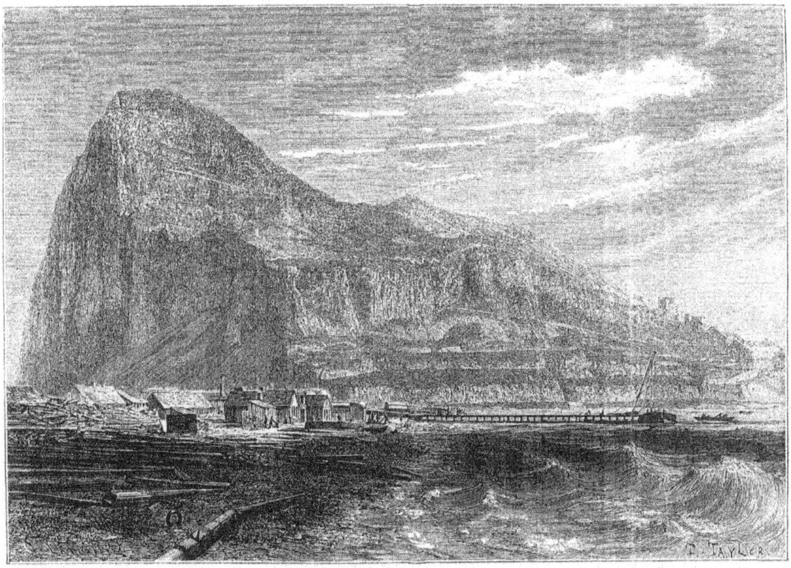

VUE DE GIBRALTAR, PRISE DE L'ISTHME DE LA LINEA.

Illustration 16 The Rock of Gibraltar towers above the Neutral Ground linking the promontory with Spain.

Source: Reclus, E., *Nouvelle Géographie Universelle* (Paris, 1876–94)

Controlling state: Britain from 1704
Situation: Southern tip of Iberian Peninsula
Sources: Bisani (1789), Brooke (c.1830), Newman (1832), Castlereagh (1842), Hutton (c.1846), Montague (1848), Baxter (1850), Brassey (1878), Maxwell (1881), Booker (2007)

Comments:
Although there are references to a lazaretto in the Neutral Ground between Gibraltar and Spain at times of epidemic, the Rock had no permanent building for quarantine. Bisani stayed aboard his ship.[99] Brooke was allowed to land after a short sail from Tangier, but the Barbary Coast was usually considered infected.[100] Newman, unluckily, was barred from landing for a day after arriving from Britain during the cholera pandemic.[101] Cholera aside, Gibraltar was always strict or Spain would have had an excuse to impose quarantine against it from political motives. This often annoyed the Royal Navy: the warship carrying Viscount Castlereagh was quarantined from the Levant because the detention period allotted at Malta had not yet expired.[102] Hutton noticed that letters and papers from his ships were received with tongs and placed in an iron box: 'had we been actually infected with the plague, more care could hardly have been taken to prevent contagion'.[103] Montague was quarantined for much the same reason as Castlereagh had been: in this instance his ship, returning to America, had not 'ridden out our quarantine term of some fifteen days at Marseilles or Malta'.[104] Baxter found that Spanish steamers between Cadiz and Marseilles called at Algeciras while French steamers on the same run called at Gibraltar, which merited them a quarantine at Malaga.[105] It was just such a reaction at Malaga which encouraged Brassey not to sail there as planned from Gibraltar and to make for Africa instead.[106] Maxwell discovered that even in 1881 quarantine niceties at Gibraltar still existed (by reason of cholera) even for a voyage from Falmouth.[107]

GIURGEVO

QS number: 20

Controlling state: Russia (nominally Wallachia)
Situation: Danube river port, left bank, now Giurgiu in Romania
Sources: Elliott (c. 1837), Spencer (1850)

Comments:
Established directly opposite the Turkish city of Rustchuk (now Ruse in Bulgaria), which Elliott was allowed to visit without quarantine on his return. If, however, he had been perceived by his guards to touch any person or animal during the excursion, it would have cost him 'a penance of ten

days quarantine'.[108] Spencer crossed to Giurgevo from Rustchuk with an Arabian horse:

> 'a Russian police officer . . . drove me and my horse before him to the sanitary room, where after we had undergone a thorough fumigation, my four-legged companion was restored to liberty, while his poor master was led captive into the presence of the military commander, for insurgent Wallachia was still under martial law.'[109]

There was much interrogation, but the quarantine formalities were over.

GUMRY

QS number: 21

Controlling state: Russia
Situation: Boundary quarantine station on the route from Erzurum in Turkey to Tiflis (now Tbilisi) in Georgia; now Gyumri in Armenia
Sources: Perkins (1834)

Comments:
Perkins referred to a 'quarantine ground' rather than 'station' and was confined to 'a hollow, on the bank of a small muddy brook' for 14 days.

> 'Six or eight dozen of geese thronged us on every side; flies, like the swarms of Egypt, flocked into our tent, to devour us and our provisions; sand, from the surrounding sun-burnt hills, sifted upon us, on every breeze; and a stench, from animals that had died during quarantine, their bodies being left unburied, annoyed us sometimes almost to suffocation.'

There were, however, quarantine buildings for the administration and a fumigation room. Perkins found the food disgusting and the behaviour of officials little better; indeed, he was 'heart-sickened' by the brutality of the Russian regime.[110]

HEBRON

QS number: 22

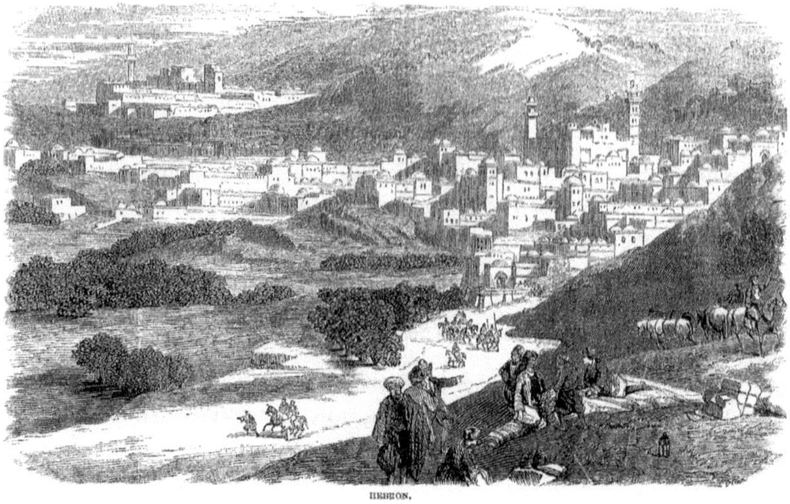

Illustration 17 The approach to Hebron in the mid-nineteenth century. The local stone, as at Gaza, was not conducive to a strong lazaretto.

Source: Thomson, W., *The Land and the Book* (New York, 1859)

Controlling state: Palestine (within Ottoman Empire)
Situation: Southwest of Jerusalem
Sources: Gadsby (1847), Monk (1848)

Comments:

Gadsby and his party arrived to find a doctor who 'lectured us severely for daring to enter the town without having received pratique' and warned that he could detain them for 15 days.[111] But the problem was quickly resolved by a payment of 100 piastres. Apparently quarantine facilities really existed, as Monk mentioned, 'The old lazaretto was tumbling to pieces, and a new one was being erected at a stone's throw from my tent'.[112] During his week of detention, Monk found the tranquility 'only broken by the monotonous sound of the masons' tools in the new lazaretto, built like all the houses of Hebron of stone'.[113]

HYDRA

QS number: 23

Controlling state: Greece
Situation: One of the Saronic Islands, off the coast of the Morea
Sources: Minet (1835), Murray (1840)

Comments:

Minet gave few details but exchanged a comfortable ship for 'the bare walls of the Quarantine establishment' and tired of it very quickly.[114] Murray wrote,

> 'Hydra has one of the best Lazarettos in Greece. It is a spacious new building, situated at Mandraki, a small and secure port one mile and a half from the town of Hydra. The rooms are good, well arranged, clean, and well ventilated. Attached to the Lazaretto is an extensive yard for exercise.'[115]

The site, however, was too far from Athens, and Hydra had minimal use, losing business first to Aegina and later to Piraeus.

JERUSALEM

QS number: 24

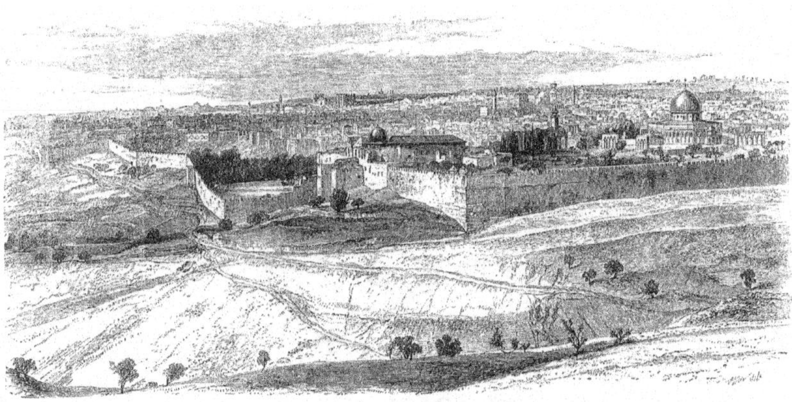

Illustration 18 The prospect of Jerusalem from near the Mount of Olives.

Source: Macleod, N., *Eastward* (London & New York, 1866)

Controlling state: Palestine (within Ottoman Empire)
Situation: Judaean Mountains
Sources: Measor (1842), Borrer (1843)

Comments:

Measor was taken aback by the requirement for quarantine, which he barely succeeded in avoiding thanks to an appeal to higher authorities. 'Where we should have passed quarantine, had they enforced it, I am at a loss to know, unless it be that they would have allowed us to encamp in some vacant place outside the city'.[116] Borrer discovered, to his cost, that the site was within it:

> 'we arrived at an open plot which seemed the public receptacle for the scrapings and off-scourings of the town, and dedicated wholly to dogs, herds of which were revelling midst heaps of canine luxuries. A low wall of rough stones surrounded this place, and in one corner was a mosque . . . [from] the old wooden door of which . . . a damp and musty smell issued forth, as if it were full of dead men's bones. Entering, we found a chamber of some thirty feet square, with a domed ceiling and walls which had originally been white, but now were green, whilst the floor was nothing more than the bare earth covered with vermin and dirt. Revolting as this was for an abiding-place, yet experience . . . taught us how sovereign a remedy is patience.'[117]

Following a visit from the British consul, they were allowed to pitch tents behind his house.

KARTAL, *SEE* CONSTANTINOPLE

KAVAK, *SEE* CONSTANTINOPLE

KULELI, *SEE* CONSTANTINOPLE

LA SPEZIA, *SEE* GENOA

LEGHORN

QS number: 25

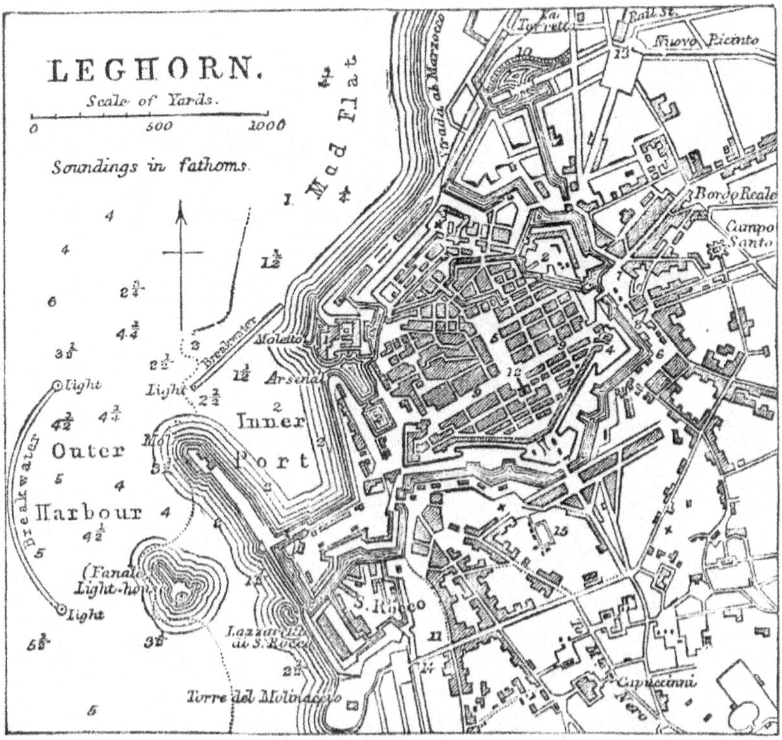

1 Fortezza Vecchia
2 Fortezza Nuova
3 Fortezza de San Pietro
4 Bastione San Cosimo
5 Piazza d'Arme
6 Piazza San Beneditto
7 Piazza Rangoni
8 Piazza dei Condotti
9 Via Ferdinanda
10 New Naval Arsenal
11 Campo di Marte or Piazza San Rocco
12 Duomo
13 Porto di San Marco
14 Nuova Porta a Mare

Illustration 19 Port of Leghorn c. 1870. This map shows only the central lazaretto of San Rocco, the earliest of three quarantine stations at this busy port.

Source: *Imperial Gazetteer* (London, Glasgow & Edinburgh, 1878)

Controlling state: Tuscany; Kingdom of Italy, 1861
Situation: Mediterranean seaport (Livorno in Italian)
Sources: Mundy (c. 1608), Fermanel (1631), Thévenot (1656), Carré (1674), Tournefort (1702), Labat (1706), de Sainte-Maure (1721), de Saumery (1724), Grosley (18th century), Prutky (1756), Ives (1758), La Lande (1765), Howard (1778), de Binos (1779), Daschkaw (c.1780), Rooke (1783), Tully (1785), Sutherland (1788), Granville (1794),

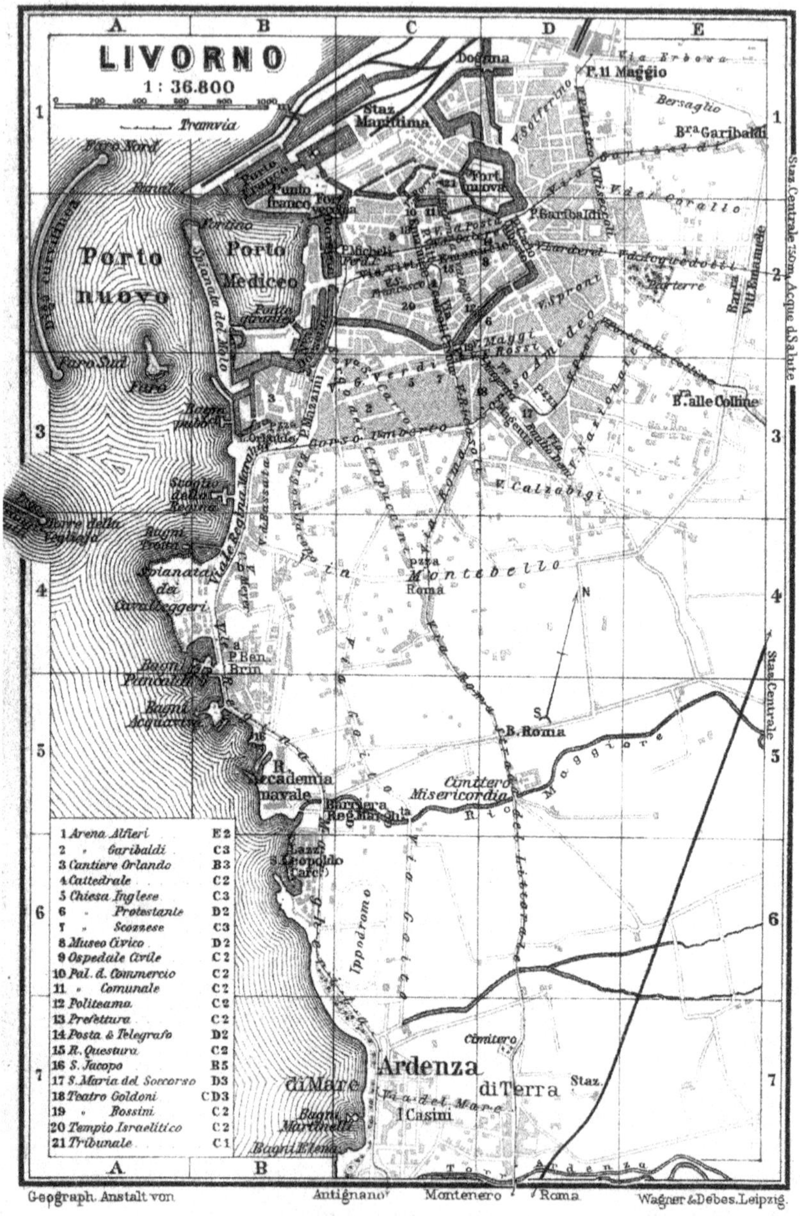

Illustration 20 The later lazarettos of Leghorn were on either side of the mouth of the Rio Maggiore, shown in the lower half of this map. The lazaretto of San Leopoldo is still named; the naval academy to the north absorbed the premises of the lazaretto San Jacopo.

Source: Baedeker, K., *Northern Italy* (Leipzig, 1913)

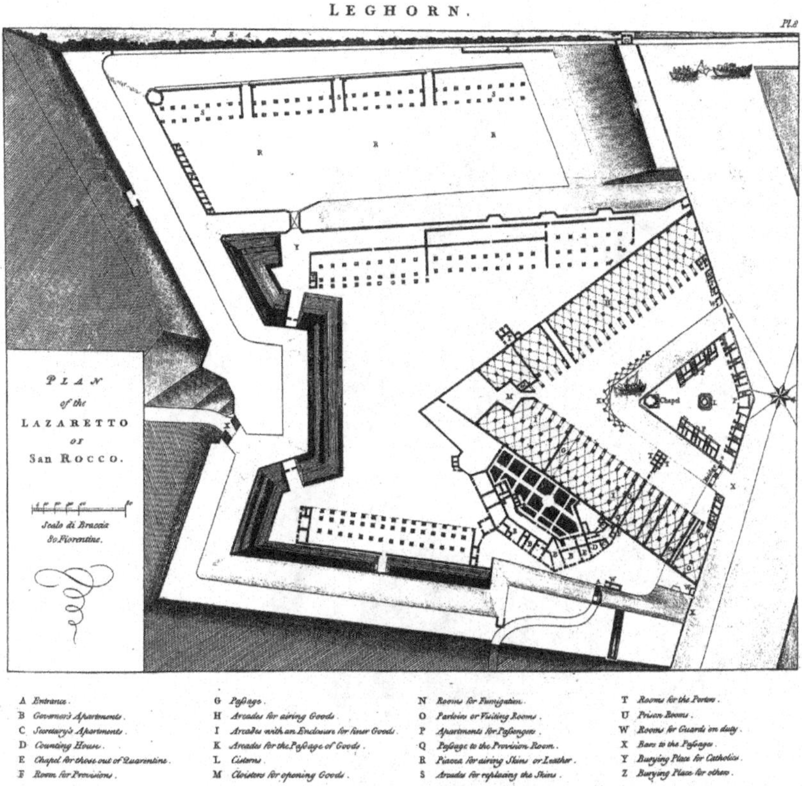

Illustration 21 Ground plan of the lazaretto of San Rocco at Leghorn.

Source: Howard, J., *An Account of the Principal Lazarettos in Europe* (London, 1791)

Macgill (1806), Semple (1806), Dodwell (1806), Bedford (1814), Matthews (1817), Strutt (1820), Sinclair (1827), Buckingham (1828), Valery (1830s), Asmar (1832), Minet (1837), Knight (1838), Fulchiron (1838), Panzac (1986)

Comments:

The best-regarded, largest and busiest quarantine station for merchandise and the natural successor to Venice. In terms of passengers, however, the port lost ground to Malta in the nineteenth century, despite having three operational lazarettos. The earliest of these, following Leghorn's free-port status in the late sixteenth century, was the lazaretto of San Rocco close to the harbour. The lazaretto of San Jacopo was built around 50 years later to the south of the port; and the lazaretto of San Leopoldo, named after Grand Duke Leopold, was under construction nearby in 1778 during the visit by

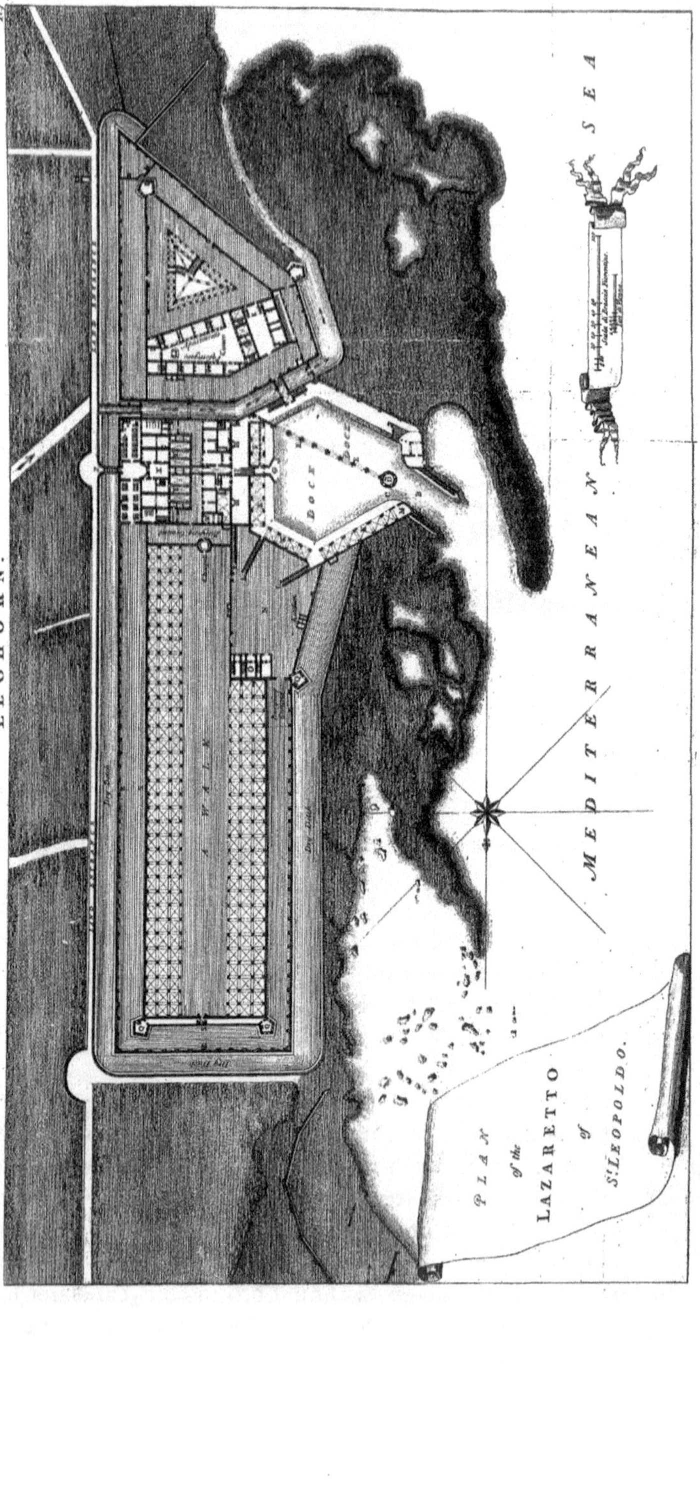

Illustration 22 Ground plan of the lazaretto of San Leopoldo at Leghorn.
Source: Howard, J., *An Account of the Principal Lazarettos in Europe* (London, 1791)

Howard, who noted 47 slaves employed there. He was impressed by the official emphasis 'on the health and convenience of the passengers' and was told by the British ambassador at Constantinople 'that the lazarettos at Leghorn are the best in Europe'.[118] Mundy mentioned 'Prattick' [pratique] there and thought the town was 'the neatest, cleanest and pleasantest place' he had ever seen.[119] Fermanel avoided quarantine from the Levant by arriving via Sicily, although he had not been allowed to enter the Sicilian port of Trapano.[120] Thévenot avoided quarantine also, to his own surprise, but his ship had captured a prize which promised immediate profit for local interests.[121] Carré was less fortunate, being taken to a lazaretto for political reasons after a brief voyage from Messina.[122] Tournefort, arriving from Smyrna, got away with only four days' quarantine.[123] None of these episodes bears out Labat's claim that rules at Leghorn were tight because the health of Europe depended on them.[124]

Not until de Saumery are there precise details of the system. He stayed aboard his ship (from Smyrna) for ten days while the cargo received a token airing, after which he was taken to the lazaretto of San Jacopo where his little group was allotted '*trois belles chambres*', of which one was adequately furnished. He chronicled in some detail his experiences in this 'prison', which he summarized as boring but not unpleasant, while recognizing that the less advantaged among the '*rapsodie de toutes sortes de gens*' had a bad time of it.[125] Grosley casually visited the lazaretto of San Rocco as a tourist, the first of several later visitors; unaware of the pitfalls, he was lucky not to be ordered into quarantine or even fired upon.[126] Prutky entered the lazaretto of San Jacopo where he 'lived comfortably enough' before being struck down by 'a very severe tertian ague'.[127] His quarantine, however, was not extended by his illness. Ives was also laid low by dysentery in a Leghorn lazaretto, but he did not specify which one. Despite anger with the authorities at the length of his quarantine, he found the behaviour of the captain of the lazaretto 'exceedingly polite'.[128]

An unusual assessment of quarantine at Leghorn was given by La Lande, who claimed that when a ship from the Levant posed too much risk, it was sent on to Marseilles. He also noted that the lazaretto of San Rocco was too close to the town and that another was being built further away.[129] It is not clear from de Binos in which lazaretto he passed his quarantine, but his companions (all strangers to each other) were so pleasant that the location did not matter.[130] Princess Daschkaw, on the other hand, was very specific, visiting 'the new hospital for performing quarantine', which was the lazaretto San Leopoldo.[131] As the Grand Duke had given orders for her reception, she was naturally left with a good impression and motivated to recommend such a building to the Russian authorities. Rooke was among those who took quarantine in their stride,[132] while Tully wrote that 'purity in quarantines' was found only at Leghorn. He believed (inaccurately) that the lazaretto San Rocco was initially the place for 'those persons actually infected with plague'; that the lazaretto San Jacopo (which he called 'St.

Jachimo') was for 'convalescents from the first'; and that the third, 'handsomest of them all', was for persons arriving with a clean bill of health from Barbary.[133]

Sutherland appears to have completed 15 days' quarantine on his ship in Leghorn Roads, while Countess Granville, coming only from Gibraltar, certainly did her three-day detention on board the ship *St. George*.[134] Macgill reckoned that the lazarettos of Leghorn were 'the finest and most commodious that can be imagined, being in an airy situation close upon the beach, and built like small fortresses, with a deep moat, and high wall around them'.[135] Semple passed his quarantine on board ship, first in the outer harbour and then within the mole. He calculated that vessels were deliberately kept from docking for mercantile reasons: by the time the masters and agents were eventually ashore they were only too pleased to sell their cargoes at the first 'plausible offer'.[136] Dodwell was caught by a political problem. He arrived at Leghorn at a time of French intrigue and was judged to be a spy. This earned him 'a quarantine of twenty-one days, in a miserable boat' with little cover. When he eventually landed, he was briefly gaoled.[137] The 6th Duke of Bedford had no complaints about his treatment in the lazaretto San Jacopo, beyond the fact that he was there at all, having arrived only from Algeciras in southern Spain. The problem was an epidemic at Gibraltar.[138]

Matthews, like Semple before him, passed his quarantine on board ship within the mole of the inner harbour.[139] Strutt was another lazaretto tourist and made the familiar mistake of treating the system too lightly so he was lucky to get out again.[140] Sinclair limited his inspection to the view of San Leopoldo from a pleasure boat.[141] The 1st Duke of Buckingham and Chandos thought all three lazarettos at Leghorn seemed 'admirably qualified for their object', and Valery thought 'the' lazaretto (probably San Rocco) was 'truly superb of its kind'.[142] Princess Asmar spent 40 days in quarantine, probably in San Leopoldo, and was startled by the strict surveillance.[143] Minet's friend Mr Hemery was also unimpressed, finding the lazaretto 'a most comfortless place'.[144] Knight did not give himself the opportunity of finding out, as he chose to remain 35 days quarantined on his ship, despite the possibility of abridging the period by going to a lazaretto.[145] Fulchiron learnt by hearsay that '*Le lazaret* [presumably San Leopoldo] *est beau, parfaitement tenu*'.[146]

San Rocco was used until 1852 and demolished around ten years later; San Jacopo became disused after 1860 and was demolished in 1877 to make way for a naval academy. San Leopoldo, following conversion to a prison, was demolished in 1913 to allow the same academy to expand.[147]

LISBON

QS number: 26

Controlling state: Portugal
Situation: Atlantic seaport
Sources: Sandwich (1739), Parbury (1838), Browne (1860s)

Comments:

Lisbon was usually bypassed by travellers returning from the Levant. It became a port of call for steam packets from the Mediterranean, but by then most people had quarantined at Malta or would stay aboard until England. Lord Sandwich found two lazarettos, one for clean-bill arrivals and the other for foul. The former was 'just without the walls of the city, in an island' connected by a drawbridge 'generally kept up' to the land. The foul lazaretto was three miles away on the seashore communicating with the city's moat by means of a canal. He mentioned that this lazaretto was armed with cannons and defended 'by a strong garrison of Germans'.[148] Parbury, who stayed aboard the Falmouth packet, observed that the Lisbon quarantine was strict.[149] Browne's steamer docked at Lisbon during a cholera scare. After an initial quarantine of three days aboard ship, the passengers were taken to the lazaretto sited 'on the opposite side of the bay, in an isolated position among the rocks, about three miles below'. After fumigation ceremonies, they

> 'were led about a quarter of a mile up a narrow and precipitous stone way into an old castle, whereof the beginning must have been long anterior to the Middle Ages. It was patched and cobbled together in every possible style of architecture, and was chiefly remarkable for its great gateway, and the formidable ramparts overlooking the bay.'

The views of Belem castle and the city were 'exceedingly fine' and the sleeping quarters, fleas apart, 'were tolerably good'.[150]

MALTA

QS number: 27

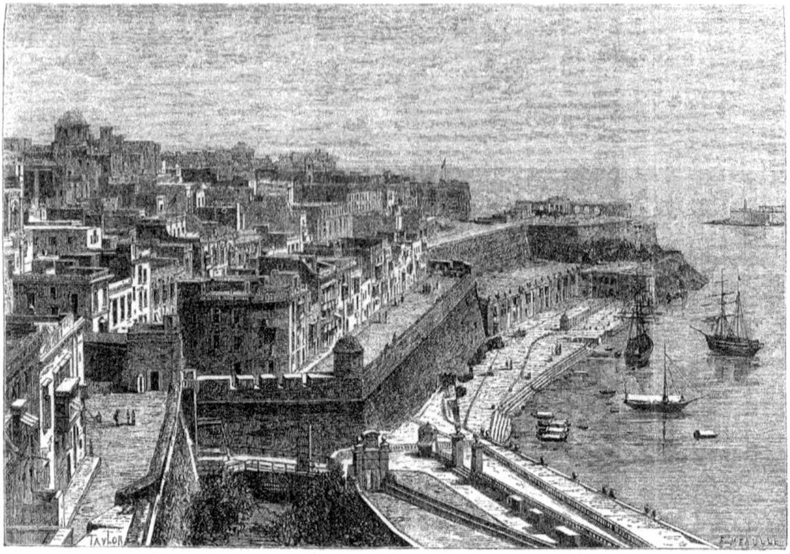

ILE DE MALTE, VUE DE LA VALETTE
Dessin de Taylor, d'après une photographie de M. Bedford.

Illustration 23 The main quay in the Grand Harbour, Valletta, where quarantine was occasionally practised until the late seventeenth century.

Source: Reclus, E., *Nouvelle Géographie Universelle* (Paris, 1876–94)

Controlling state: Order of St John of Jerusalem; France from 1798; Britain from 1800

Situation: Mediterranean island

Sources: de Beaveau (1604), Sandys (c.1610), della Valle (1625), Teonge (1675), Dumont (1690), Sainte-Maure (1721), de Saumery (1724), Sandwich (1739), Brydone (1770), Denon (1778), Howard (1785), D'Irumberry (1791), Gell (1804), Macgill (1806), Byron (1811), Cazenove (1811), Buckingham (1813), Fitzclarence (1818), Woods (1818), Rennie (1821), Strutt (1821), Wolff (1822), Sherer (1823), Hay (1824), Montefiore (1827), Malcolm (1827), Frankland (1828), Lushington (1828), Woodruff (1828), Disraeli (1830), Keppel (1830), Wilson (1830s), Slade (1830s), Scott (1831), Newman (1832–3), Waring (1833), Rochfort Scott (1833), Auldjo (1833), Fitzmaurice (1833), Giraudeau (1833), Marchebeus (1833), de Gérambe (1833), D'Estourmel (1833), Perkins (1833), de Marmont (1835), Macbrair (1835), Minet (1835), Cornille (c. 1835), Strickland (1836), Austin (1836), Meerza (1836), Minet (1837), Wilde

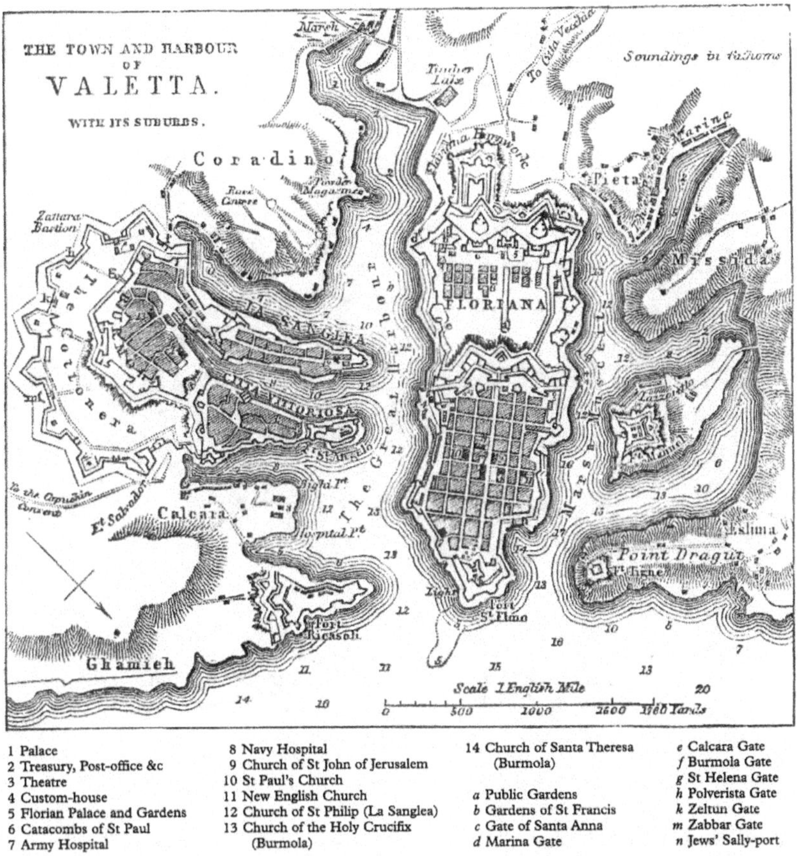

Illustration 24 Malta, c. 1870. This map shows just how many creeks and harbours constituted the port of Valletta. The lazaretto and Fort Manoel are on the island within Marsamxett Harbour to the right.

Source: *Imperial Gazetteer* (London, Glasgow & Edinburgh, 1878)

(1838), Holroyd (1838), Robertson (1838), Padbury (1838), Usborne (1839), Montefiore (1839–40), Roberts (1839), MacGill (1839), de Salle (1839), Kinnear (1839), Fane (1840), Murray, 1840), Damer (1840), Beswick (1840), Holthaus (1840), Londonderry (1841), Snow (1841), Grosvenor (1841), Angas (1841), Millard (1841), Stent (1842), Wilkinson (1843), Hervey (1843–4), Thackeray (1844), Griffith (1844), de Malherbe (1844), Murdoch (1844), Terry (1845), Wolff (1845), Watson (1845), Ampère (1845), Montauban (c.1845), Hutton (c. 1846), Beldam (1846), Young (1847), Wilkinson (1847), Gadsby (1847), Bevan (c. 1847), Montague (1848), de Gasparin (1848), Smith (1849), Pridham (1849), Baxter

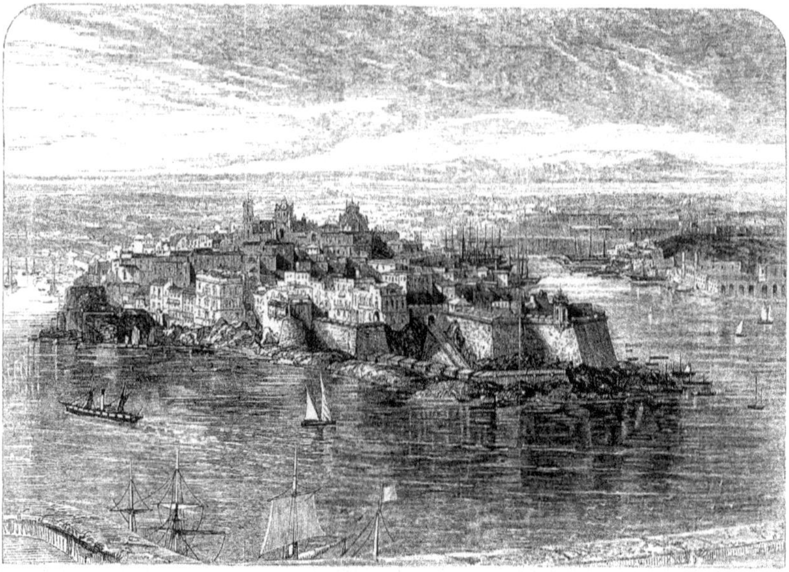

Illustration 25 A capricious view of the main harbours of Valletta in the mid-nineteenth century. The buildings on the extreme right (invisible from the assumed viewpoint) represent the lazaretto.

Source: Macleod, N., *Eastward* (London & New York, 1866)

(1849), Taylor (1852), Murray (1854), Beamont (1854), Carlisle (1854), Bussolin (1881), Cassar (1965), Panzac (1986), Booker (2007)

Comments:

Quarantine was at Valletta, whose magnificent natural setting encompassed two main anchorages, the Grand Harbour and Marsamxett Harbour. The latter was developed as a quarantine station by the Knights of St John (who had also tolerated quarantine in the Grand Harbour), and a lazaretto was built in 1666 on a peninsula (later an island) within the harbour.[151] The earliest seventeenth-century references to quarantine at Malta mentioned only precautions and concessions, and when Teonge referred to the 'Lazaretta' he meant a hospital 'under their outermost wall' for those actually infected by plague.[152] An early reference to a lazaretto on the 'little Island' came with Dumont, in 1690,[153] but most eighteenth-century travellers wrote only of concessions, staying aboard their ship, or quarantine avoidance. Howard mentioned that the lazaretto peninsula contained also Fort Manoel, which 50 years later became widely used to accommodate the quarantine overflow. As for the lazaretto itself, Howard described it as 'less airy' than the Fort, with the old part containing 16 rooms on two floors,

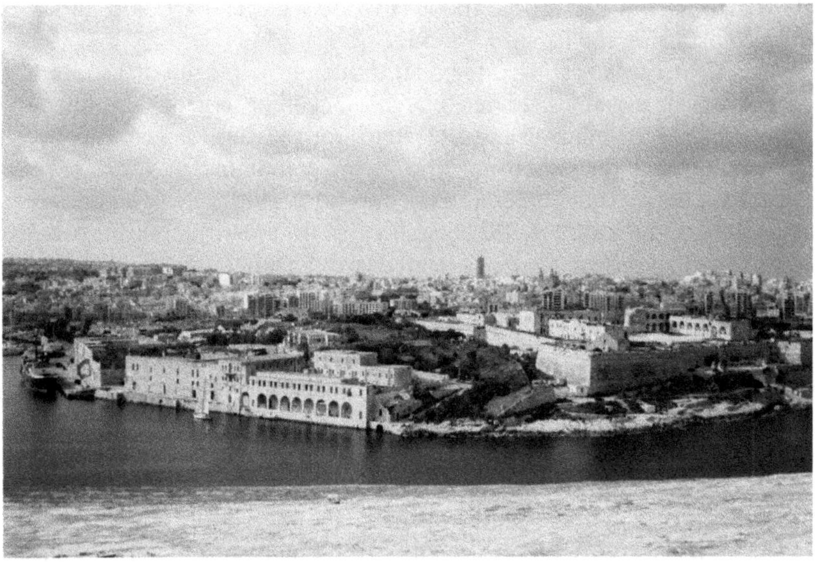

Illustration 26 A modern view of the lazaretto buildings of Malta, taken from Floriana.
Source: photograph by the author

the upper ones with balconies, while the newer part was 'more convenient for passengers, and airy for merchandise' with two courts, each 101 feet × 63 feet. The chapel was then being built near the existing burial ground.[154]

The facilities at Malta, when fully developed, were more akin to a compulsory hotel than a prison, and relatively few travellers found grounds for serious complaint. Indeed, the accolade for best environment, although occasionally contended by Leghorn and Marseilles, was undoubtedly won by Malta. Of course, there were also detractors. Persons on their own, like D'Irumberry, could find their room '*vaste et solitaire*', while the temperament of Byron would have been ruffled by any confinement.[155] Cazenove found 'two fine large rooms . . . in a stone building of large dimensions, but bare as a rock'.[156] This absence of basic furnishings was eventually remedied by the authorities, but extra furniture was always needed and could be hired or bought from Valletta. Woods liked his two rooms (each 27 feet square and nearly 20 feet high), which were supplemented by a vaulted gallery 120 feet long and a terrace of similar length.[157] For Sherer, however, the 'spacious and cool' apartments were not quite enough, as the gallery and terrace did not make up for the absence of an exercise yard.[158] Mrs Lushington made a similar point five years later.[159] Lady Montefiore explained that her party did quarantine at the palace, 'the larger part of the building of the lazaretto being so denominated'. Indeed, she thought the rooms were palatial 'though not on account of their decorations; but they are perfectly clean and agreeably situated'.[160] This 'palace' was probably what the authorities referred to as the Palazzo Grande (Howard's newer part), the older and smaller part being the Palazzo Vecchio.

Fort Manoel was first used for quarantine in the plague of 1813 and re-entered regular use about 15 years later. MacGill observed, 'This fine fort is at present [1839] employed as a Lazzaretto for passengers: the influx becoming so great, since the establishment of steam communication, that the regular Lazzaretto, was unequal to their depuration'.[161] Mrs Lushington thought it was where 'the military and persons of rank under quarantine are quartered',[162] but a lot depended on preference and availability. Auldjo recorded that his prestigious party had a choice between the lazaretto proper and the Fort: 'the latter for the Prince, and such as chose to go there in preference to the former'.[163] In the case of many travellers, such as Disraeli, it is not clear exactly where they were quarantined as the term 'lazaretto' was loosely applied to both buildings. Sir Walter Scott is a particular problem, having been quarantined in 'the decayed chambers of a magnificent old Spanish palace', apparently representing an exceptional concession within the town.[164]

Newman, on the other hand, was most specific and orthodox. Not only was he in the lazaretto, but he described it minutely, beginning with the gallery which ran around the outside wall, halfway up. He thought the rooms generally were 'fine', at least 50 feet × 30 feet with an arched roof and whitewashed walls. He and his companion occupied four rooms and a kitchen, and he sketched the layout in a letter.[165] Newman counted himself lucky to have a fireplace as he believed there was only one other in the building. Certainly Frankland, four years earlier, had lamented the absence of fireplaces in 'the lazaretto quarters'.[166] This is curious as Wilkinson's guidebook mentioned that rooms in the lazaretto 'have the comfort of fire-places',[167] and Waring noted that his room *did* have a fireplace. Waring is useful more generally for pinpointing the layout of the lazaretto: there was 'a square court in the middle, from which a wide flight of steps ascends to an open gallery running all round, and communicating with the different apartments. The ground-floor is used for warehouses, fumigating-rooms, and other offices'. He described the apartment allocated to himself and his companion as 'an immense dismal place, forty-three feet long, twenty-six broad, and about twenty feet high, with the roof supported upon arches'.[168] The walls of the lazaretto, he noted, were ten feet thick, prompting Marchebeus to remark that '*rien n'a été épargné pour la solidité de sa construction*', but he found the arrangement '*privé de courant d'air*'.[169]

Eusèbe de Salle commented favourably on the rooms at Fort Manoel, which he found clean, spacious and airy, with a view over both harbours and the open sea.[170] Kinnear went into more detail about the Fort's accommodation: 'I have two sitting-rooms and a very comfortable sleeping apartment above, with every sort of convenience' and 'a tolerable space of the ramparts to walk on'.[171] Mrs Damer found that the governor of Malta himself had secured for her party 'the most comfortable quarters' in Fort Manoel.[172] Beswick, also, would have wished to stay in the Fort, but it was full; Lady Londonderry was equally unhappy to be in the lazaretto itself.[173] Mrs Griffith was anxious to be in the Fort in July as it was considered the cooler location, 'but there was no good room vacant'.[174] The attractions of the Fort were summed up by de Malherbe, who called it '*un magnifique lazaret, admirablement bien exposé, et dans lequel on jouit d'une assez grande liberté et d'une existence fort supportable*'.[175]

But if the lazaretto itself seemed a less welcome destination, it was better equipped. Murray advised that all rooms there were 'large, and to each set a kitchen is attached; a provision boat arrives morning and evening'.[176] Some of these kitchens became redundant after 1838 when the lazaretto acquired its own *trattoria*, which, as Snow discovered, also sent meals to the Fort.[177] Stent reckoned that Malta provided quarantine 'conveniences of even a luxurious description',[178] and Wilkinson was almost as enthusiastic: 'the rooms are good, the facilities of obtaining every requisite great, and more privileges are accorded with fewer vexations than in other lazarettos'.[179] But such praise did not prevent Hervey turning his nose up at the prospect of the lazaretto or deter Thackeray from being sarcastic about the regime at Fort Manoel, where the authorities were 'so careful of your health as to lock you up in your room every night'.[180] And Mrs Griffith bemoaned that her three rooms (and a kitchen) in the lazaretto were completely unfurnished, even in 1844, while Mrs Montauban thought the 'restaurant within the building' supplied 'indifferent fare'.[181] Bevan would have agreed with that: he went 'to the common-hall' at the sound of the dinner bell, and found that his 4 shillings and 6 pence bought only a 'low diet, such as weak broth with salads and sour-krout, and no end of gherkins and beet-root'.[182]

Despite the refurbishment of the lazaretto in the 1830s, most travellers still preferred the Fort, which made it impossible over many decades for the authorities to restore it to the military. In 1847 for instance, Young felt 'some regret at the idea of being cooped up for twelve days in the lazaretto, the more so as we found that Fort Manoel was not our destination'.[183] Wilkinson's guidebook of the same year could have influenced Young's thinking, as he wrote, 'There are two lazarettos at Malta. That of Fort Manoel is by far the most comfortable'.[184] Bevan reported that it was subdivided into three separate buildings, each capable of accommodating from 12 to 20 persons, and one being exclusively for the sick.[185] The plaudits continued for Malta, with Smith's simple testimonial that 'the lazaretto is the best of its kind' being typical of many.[186] But as the nineteenth century progressed, and the principle of quarantine passed out of fashion, so the niggling imperfections gained ground. Baxter summed up the mood in 1849: there was nothing any longer to 'justify the plan of putting people into rooms without glass windows, with stone uncovered floors, and a mere stick of furniture'.[187] It was not surprising, therefore, that some of the later quarantine detainees remained on their ships.

It was 1939 before the lazaretto finally broke all sanitary links, falling under the wing of Fort Manoel, which had long been restored to military use.[188] Both buildings suffered heavily in World War II, but much of the lazaretto is still visible today. There are very welcome plans for its restoration.

MARSEILLES

QS number: 28

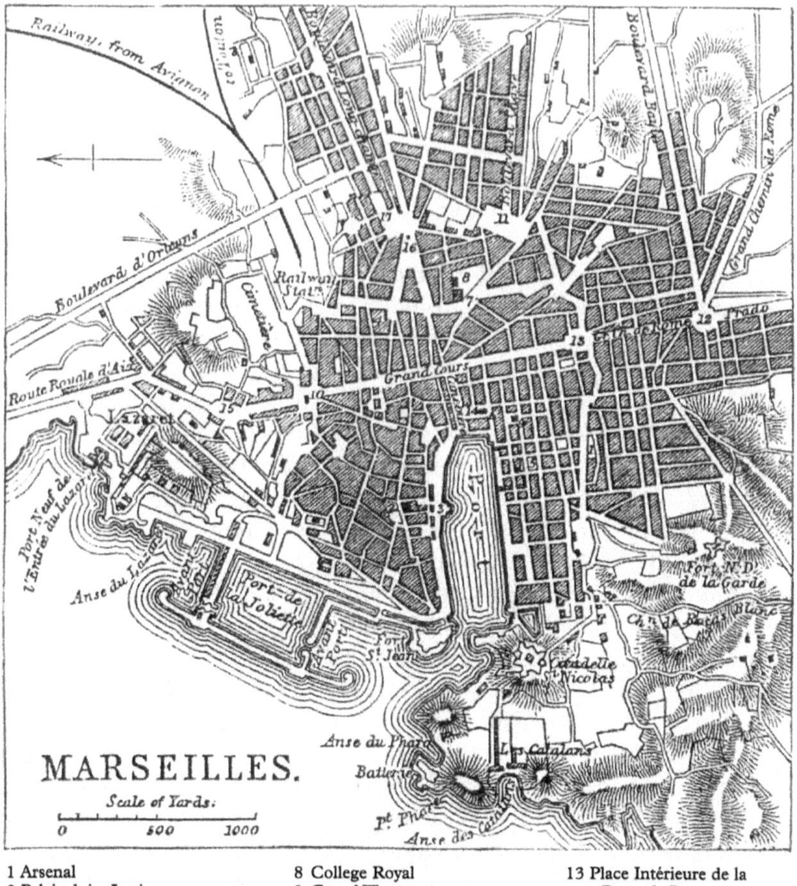

1 Arsenal
2 Palais duite Justice
3 Hotel de Ville
4 Hotel des Monnaies
5 Hotel des Douanes
6 Bourse
7 Musée et Bibliothèque
8 College Royal
9 Grand Theatre
10 Arc de Triomphe
11 Plaine de St Michael (Champ de Mars)
12 Place Castelane
13 Place Intérieure de la Porte de Rome
14 Place Royale
15 Place Pentagone
16 Fontaine Beauveau
17 Cours du Chapitre

Illustration 27 Port of Marseilles c. 1870. The 'Lazaret' with its own small harbour is shown on the outskirts of the town towards the north.

Source: *Imperial Gazetteer* (London, Glasgow & Edinburgh, 1878)

Controlling state: France
Situation: Mediterranean seaport
Sources: Carré (1674), Daniel (1701), Comelin (1720), Plaisted (1750), Howard (1785), Grellet (1807), Trant (1815), Pouqueville (1816), Meryon (1817), Irby & Mangles (1818), de Forbin (1818), van Tets

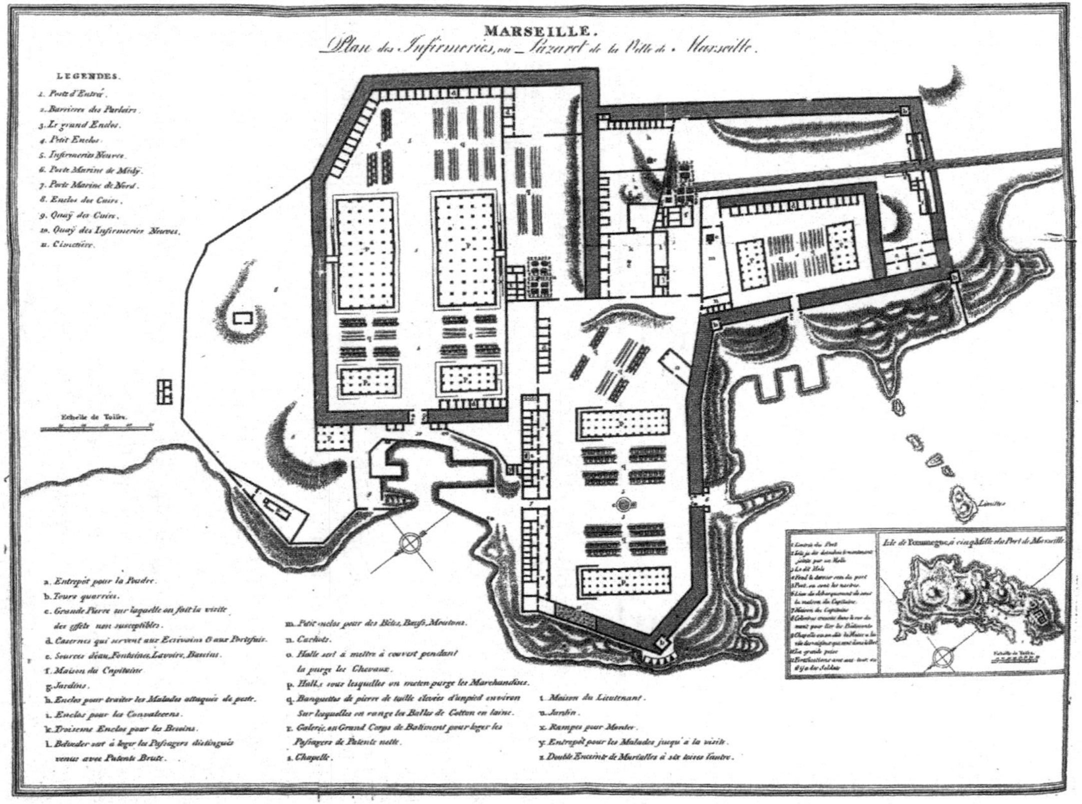

Illustration 28 Ground plan of the lazaretto at Marseilles.

Source: Howard, J., *An Account of the Principal Lazarettos in Europe* (London, 1791)

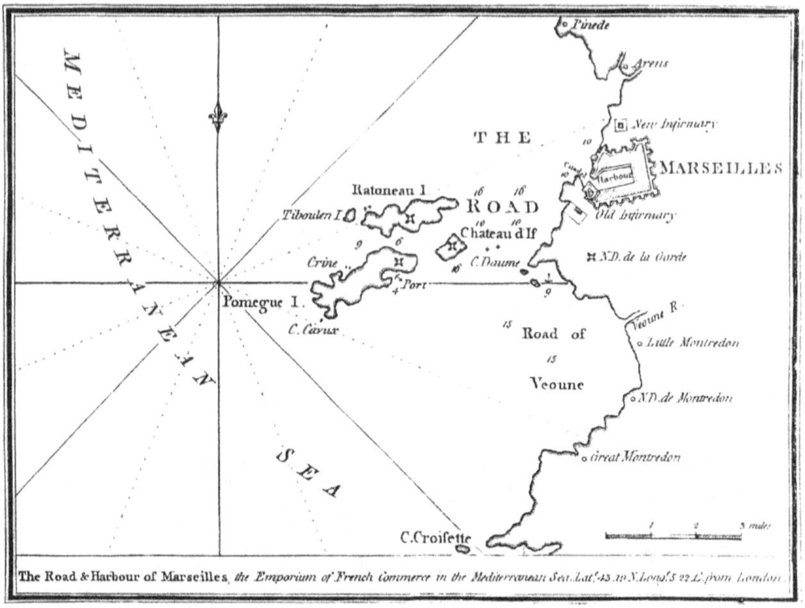

Illustration 29 The main islands off Marseilles were used for the inspection of ships with foul bills. Notice also the Old and New Infirmaries on either side of the city. The New Infirmary developed into the major lazaretto.

Source: *Naval Chronicle* (1817)

(1819), Damoiseau (1820), Malcolm (1828), Starke (1828), Stendhal (1830s), Rockwell (1835), Pardoe (1835), Demidoff (1837), Romer (1842), Wilkinson (1843), Galton (1845), Montague (1848), de Gasparin (1848), Panzac (1986)

Comments:

Details of the earliest lazaretto are obscure, but the second, known as *les vieilles infirmeries*, was built in the mid-sixteenth century to the south of the town, in an area which became known as Les Catalans.[189] The third lazaretto, known as *les nouvelles infirmeries*, was built well to the north in the 1660s.[190] A smart health office was erected on the northern quay of *le vieux port* in around 1720, and it still exists today in other usage. Certain islands near the mouth of the port, especially Pomègues, were also used for quarantine purposes. Procedures were sometimes slack before the horrific plague of 1720, which spread from causes that quarantine was specifically there to prevent. As an example of slackness, Carré was allowed ashore immediately by pleading urgent business at court.[191] Daniel, on the

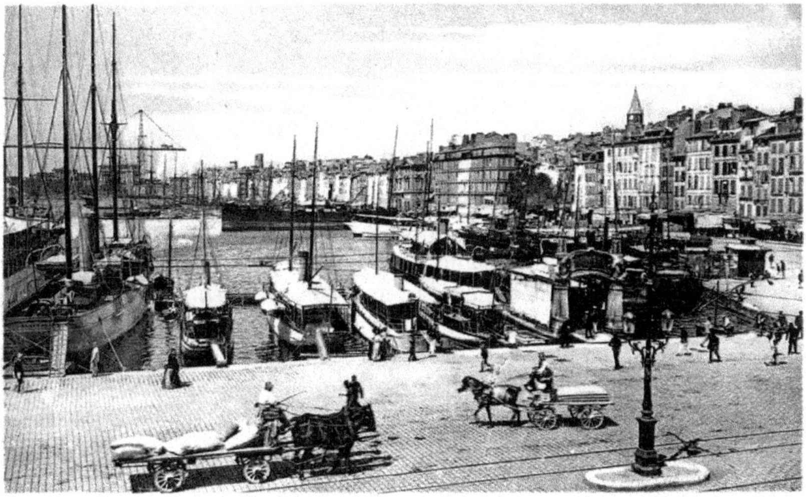

13. - MARSEILLE. - Le Vieux Port

Illustration 30 The *Vieux Port* of Marseilles around 1905. The old health office is at the end of the right-hand quay, close to the transporter bridge (long demolished) glimpsed in the distance.

Source: postcard

other hand, suffered a full 40 days, although Comelin, returning from North Africa with freed slaves, was excused any quarantine as the voyage had been nearly two months.[192] Plaisted found 'very convenient' rooms in the lazaretto, arranged 'ten in a Row' behind a gallery stretching for 225 feet. The rooms were numbered, and when a visitor arrived from town to converse with a detainee at the *parlatorio*, the gatekeeper tolled a bell as many times as the number of the room. The circumference of the whole lazaretto was about a mile. Plaisted had satisfactory dinners provided from an internal caterer, although it was possible (and cheaper) to order from the town.[193] Howard inspected the lazaretto closely and reproduced a plan in his book. 'Among other apartments for passengers', he wrote, 'there are twenty-four large rooms, of which some are above stairs, and open into a spacious gallery enclosed by lattice'. Facilities included a chapel and 'a tavern' which supplied 'dinners and suppers' and had 'the exclusive privilege of supplying . . . wine'.[194] This was evidently from where Plaisted had been served. Grellet described the lazaretto as 'very airy' and 'divided into several blocks' with 'spacious yards', but he would have liked more furniture than a table, two chairs and an iron bedstead.[195]

Clarissa Trant, confusing matters, placed the lazaretto near Fort St Jean and compared it to 'a little English Village' on account of the small white houses.[196] Not until Henrica van Tets are there any further descriptions of the site: she was alluding to the traditional '*grand établissement au bord de la mer*', but she used language similar to Trant's in that she likened the interior of the lazaretto to '*une petite ville*' containing bakers, butchers and cooks.[197] Damoiseau arrived there with Arabian horses, which exercised in the grounds to recover from the voyage.[198] Malcolm was struck both by the 'absurdly minute quarantine regulations' and by the obnoxiously real painting in the health office of plague sufferers.[199] Starke explained that this painting was by David and deemed the lazaretto to be the best in Europe.[200] Stendhal thought the painting (and a companion piece) were by Serre (which they were), and he described the lazaretto as '*un vaste édifice qui se prolonge depuis la pointe de la Joliette jusqu'à la pointe d'Arenc*'. Stendhal noticed seven enclosures, four for people and three for goods. He was impressed by the double perimeter walls, 25 feet high and 36 feet apart, the gap being regularly patrolled.[201] Rockwell liked them too, calling the lazaretto 'one of the most beautiful and secure in the world', covering a space 'one fifteenth of that occupied by the whole city'.[202]

Julia Pardoe had no inclination to describe the lazaretto, having been trapped and terrified nearby at a time of virulent cholera: her place of quarantine was her lodging house.[203] The port was calm again when Demidoff was quarantined, and he found the repose rather welcome.[204] For Isabella Romer, the health office on the quay was the main attraction, especially the paintings about plague and cholera: she was another who cited the main painting as a work by David and described it as '*horriblement beau*!'[205] Wilkinson called it 'alarmingly striking' but, despite its message, thought the quarantine at Marseilles was 'unnecessarily scrupulous'.[206] Galton caused havoc in the lazaretto when one of his pet monkeys got loose and scampered around everywhere, causing his guardian to be 'transported with rage'.[207] Montague managed to perform quarantine on his ship.[208] Madame de Gasparin was one of the last to experience the lazaretto and described it as on a little mound covered with lavender and broom, which predisposed her to such a comfortable stay that she almost got a taste for imprisonment, even if the décor was faded and the soft furnishings often in tatters.[209] Within a few months, quarantine, as far as it was practised at all, moved to the Caroline Hospital built nearly 30 years earlier on the island of Ratonneau, and the lazaretto proper was overrun by the docks of La Joliette.[210]

MESSINA
QS number: 29

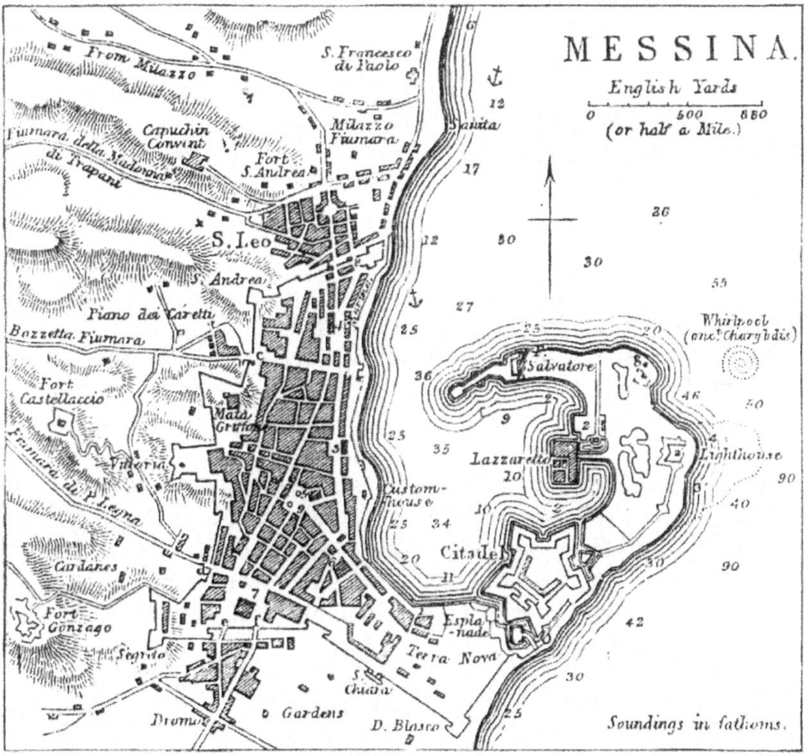

1 Arsenal
2 Flotilla Arsenal
3 Senate House
4 New Palace
5 Cathedral
6 Archbishop's Palace
7 Hospital
8 Theatre
9 The Piazza
a Porta Reale
b Porta Ferdinanda
c Porta Bocetta
d Porta Legna
e Porta Vecchia
f Porta Nuova
g Inner Light

Illustration 31 Port of Messina c. 1870. Virtually an island, the lazaretto is clearly marked on the eastern side of the harbour, while the health office (*Sanita*) is shown to the north of the town.

Source: *Imperial Gazetteer* (London, Glasgow & Edinburgh, 1878)

Controlling state: Sicily; Naples (Kingdom of the Two Sicilies) from 1816
Situation: Mediterranean seaport
Sources: Lucas (1703), Labat (1720), Pococke (1740), Nugent (1749), Brydone (1770), Howard (1785), Sutherland (1788), Queen Caroline (c. 1816)

Comments:
The lazaretto built on an island in the harbour was praised by Lucas as '*un des plus beaux & des plus commodes que j'aye vûs*'.[211] Labat found it

so full of people and merchandise that it overflowed into huts on shore.[212] Pococke thought it 'very convenient . . . on an island now divided into three parts by artificial canals, the whole being built round a large court', a form of words largely borrowed by Nugent.[213] Howard published a ground plan and elevations.[214] Following the devastating plague of 1743, sanitary measures at Messina were tightened, and even 45 years later ships from infected ports were not permitted to dock.[215] Queen Caroline expected to land there without quarantine from North Africa, but pratique was refused and she sailed on to Italy.[216]

MOZDOK

QS number: 30

Controlling state: Russia
Situation: Caucasus, at the crossing of River Terek from Georgia
Sources: Lumsden (1820)

Comments:

'The quarantine consists of many houses adjoining each other, in a fine airy situation on the banks of the Terek' just over half-a-mile from Mozdok. Lumsden found that all his clothes (other than those he was wearing) and possessions were fumigated in a locked building of which, unusually, he was given the key. He was provided with palatable local wine which reminded him of champagne.[217]

NAPLES

QS number: 31

Controlling state: Kingdom of Naples (later Kingdom of the Two Sicilies)
Situation: Mediterranean seaport
Sources: Howard (1785), Swan (1824), Buckingham (1828), Cooper (1829), Scott (1831), Minet (1835), Grosvenor (1841), Senior (1851), Twain (1867), Panzac (1986)

Comments:

'The lazaretto at Naples is very small, and I am informed that too little attention is paid there to passengers and shipping, under quarantine'.[218] Thus wrote Howard, who decided to illustrate only the health office. The lazaretto itself was on the island of Nisida, in the Gulf of Pozzuoli. Panzac (in 1986) described it as a prison for young offenders.[219] In the age of sail, Naples was not on any sea route for travellers returning from the Levant, but as the nineteenth century progressed it was included in steamer schedules to and from Marseilles and was visited by yachts. Swan arrived from Malta on a British warship which was quarantined briefly in Naples

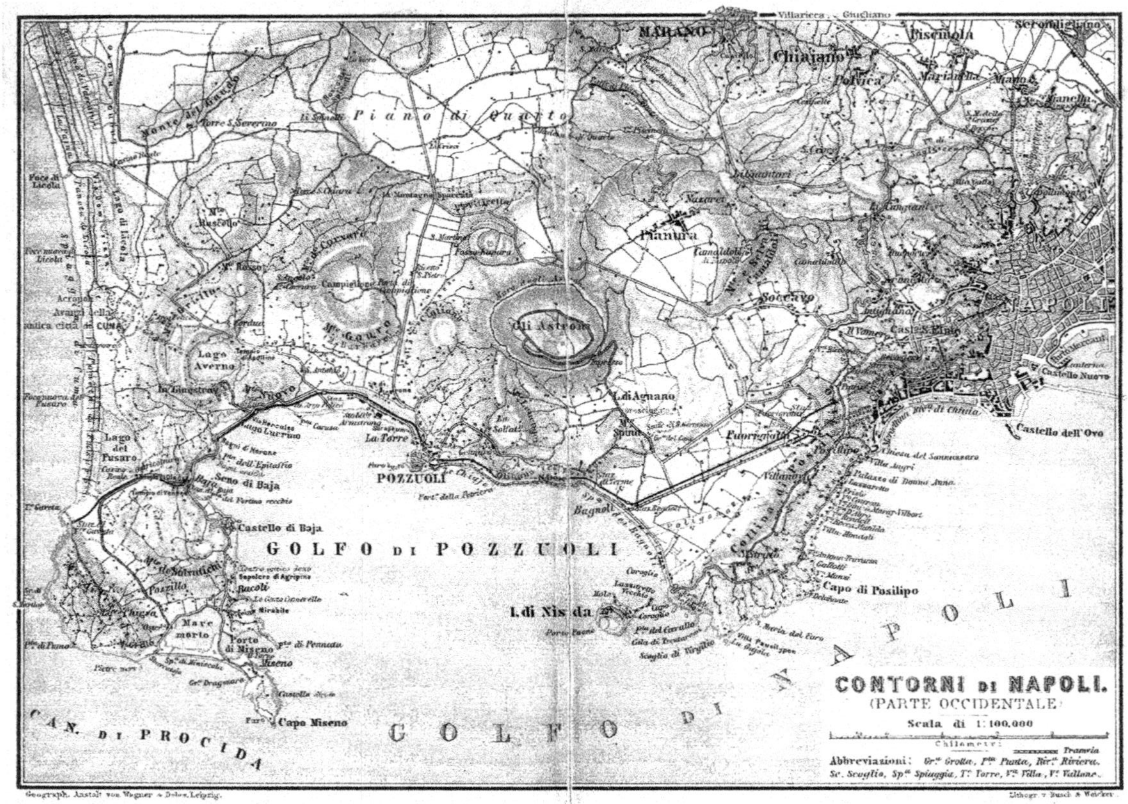

Illustration 32 The quarantine station for Naples was on the island of Nisida in the Gulf of Pozzuoli. The 'Lazzaretto Vecchio' is still shown on this map from around 1900.

Source: Baedeker, K., *Italy from the Alps to Naples* (Leipzig, 1904)

Bay.[220] The 1st Duke of Buckingham and Chandos was kept out of port for a few days under a political quarantine, as he was suspected of a link with dissidents in Calabria.[221] Cooper was among those who discovered the Neapolitan anomaly whereby the city could be approached overland without quarantine, while restrictions were enforced on arrivals by sea from elsewhere in Italy, even from Elba.[222] A more famous denouncer of this nonsense was Mark Twain, as late as 1867.[223] Sir Walter Scott was one of the few visitors by sea to have quarantine abridged, in his case by the King.[224] Lady Grosvenor's party struggled for any concession through the influence of the British ambassador.[225] Minet learnt that quarantine against cholera prevented steamers from Marseilles from getting closer to Naples than Genoa.[226] Neapolitan quarantine was notoriously fickle, which many travellers, like Senior, attributed to political motives.[227] The Privy Council in London was frequently exasperated by what it considered irrational quarantine against British shipping.

ODESSA
QS number: 32

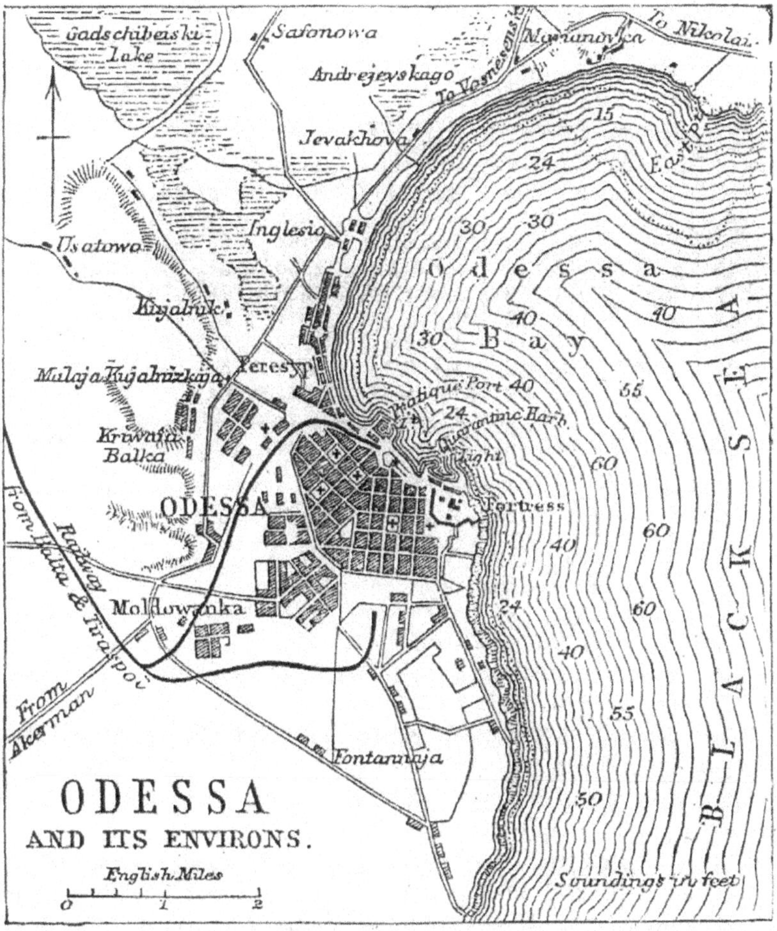

Illustration 33 Port of Odessa c. 1870, showing both the health office ('Pratique Port') and the Quarantine Harbour.

Source: *Imperial Gazetteer* (London, Glasgow & Edinburgh, 1878)

Controlling state: Russia
Situation: Black Sea seaport
Sources: Reuilly (1803), Macgill (1804, 1806), Pinkerton (1819), Moore (1824), Marmont (1834), Craven (1835), Lord de Ros (1835), Stephens (1835), Spencer (1836), Stuart (1836), Macintosh (1837), Hommaire de Hell (1838), Knight (1838), Bowring (1838), Slade (1838), Jesse (1839),

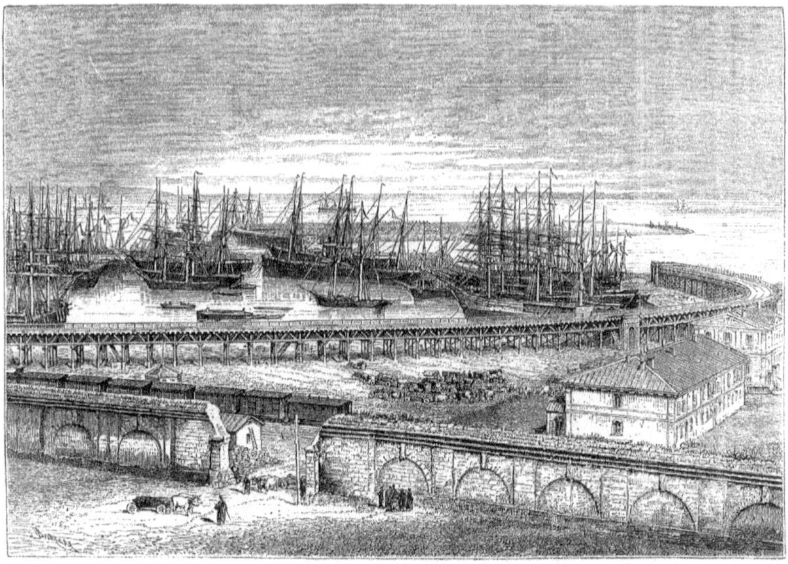

PORT D'ODESSA
Dessin de Barclay.

Illustration 34 Ships moored in Odessa Harbour in the late nineteenth century. This was more or less the view from the lazaretto.

Source: Reclus, E., *Nouvelle Géographie Universelle* (Paris, 1876–94)

Terry (1846), Pfeiffer (1848), Scott (1850), Brooks (1853), M'Culloch (1882)

Comments:

Reuilly described the inadequacies of the original lazaretto, which was no more than a collection of open sheds, formerly a barracks, behind a low stone wall and a fence. He also mentioned that the Duke de Richelieu, the Governor General of what was then New Russia, was planning a modern lazaretto on the site of an outdated fortress.[228] In August 1804, Macgill confirmed there was 'building with incredible rapidity a most spacious lazaretto' near a new mole for the harbour. In 1806, the same author called the new lazaretto 'tolerably good'.[229] Pinkerton described the site as 'half a mile above the port' consisting 'of a row of thirteen small stone apartments, one story high', five approached from the north, six from the south, and one at each end. His 'cell' was 16 feet × 13 feet and 10 feet high, with two windows, each 4 feet × 2 feet. 'A common Russian oven, made of brick-work, in one corner, with two dirty bedsteads, and a fir table three feet by two, composed the furniture'. He lived off soup, boiled meat, and tea.[230] Moore commented, as Reuilly had done, on the bad state of the original building which Richelieu superseded.[231]

Marmont eulogized the '*magnifique*' lazaretto for which he gave credit to the then Governor-General, Count Woronzow.[232] Pauline Craven also used the adjective 'magnificent' and added, 'We are here in the Lazaretto, exactly as in a pretty country house'.[233] Lord de Ros was scarcely less polite. The *spoglio* was vexing but not the accommodation:

> 'we . . . were conducted to a part of the Lazaretto where comfortable clean apartments, neatly furnished, were provided, with a sort of garden and walk in front looking over the sea, from a broken cliff, about the height of those of Ramsgate.'[234]

Stephens was struck by the beauty of the site: 'if it had not been called by that name [lazaretto] . . . we should have considered it a beautiful spot'. He described it as an enclosure of 15 to 20 acres on high ground, 'laid out in lawns and gravel walks, and ornamented with rows of acacia-trees'. The apartments were in a long row facing the sea, each with a little courtyard in front.[235] Spencer was equally impressed:

> 'The quarantine establishment is altogether well conducted. The situation, on the summit of a chain of small hills, is not only healthy but pleasant. . . . The different suites of apartments are so extensive, as almost to form a little town; each separate tenement has its small court planted with acacias: besides this, we had a public promenade, a restaurant, and a conversation-room.'[236]

Stuart commented: 'We inhabit a comfortable house; the paper and furniture of some of the rooms are really smart. I only wish that fireplaces were substituted for the high dull stoves which fill a corner of each apartment'.[237]

The ability to move around the grounds was the main attraction for Hommaire de Hell:

> 'On one of the angles of the rock there is a little platform, with seats and trees, looking down on the sea, the harbour, and part of the town. In this delightful lounging-place we often passed hours together, in contemplating the beautiful spectacle before us.'[238]

But others were less impressed. Knight called quarantine at Odessa 'disgusting', and Bowring noted that plague had 'not long ago' broken out in the lazaretto and spread to the town.[239] Slade's view was so coloured by his shambolic reception and the ignominy of his *spoglio* that he 'never passed a much more unhappy fortnight'. Yet he admitted that his apartment 'of two rooms and an ante-room' was 'good'.[240] Jesse was indignant for the same reasons as Slade but found no comfort in his apartment, despite its earlier occupation as part of Lord Durham's suite. He saw only the 'strong iron wire net work' and the 'gratings' of the doors, and even the view was little solace.[241] Terry had far more to complain about: he arrived at a crowded period in late December when the temperature was minus 18 degrees Fahrenheit, and for several nights he slept on benches trying to avoid the snoring and smoking of his unwanted Russian roommates.[242] Scott avoided quarantine but visited the lazaretto as a tourist and found it 'rather amusing', if like a zoo. Much like Jesse, he was fascinated by 'three partitions of grating' between detainees and the public.[243] Brooks was another lazaretto tourist at Odessa, quarantine being 'one of the most curious features of the place, and it is one to which the resident earliest conducts the stranger, whether the visit of the latter be for purposes of amusement or of commerce'.[244] Evidently most of the detainees were ships' crews who largely stayed on board, reaching the lazaretto only to exercise and transact business through the wires and bars of the decaying promenade.

Quarantine at Odessa was slow to decline. As late as 1882 it was noted, 'There is a convenient lazaretto, on the model of that of Marseilles'.[245]

ORSOVA, OLD

QS number: 33

Fig. 54.—The "Iron Gate."

Scale 1 : 100,000.

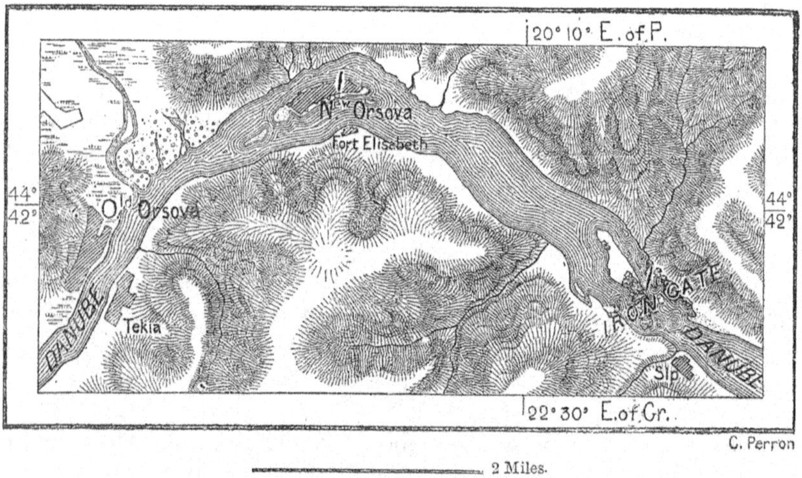

Illustration 35 Map showing the relative positions of Old and New Orsova and the infamous Iron Gate rapids downstream.

Source: Reclus, E., *Nouvelle Géographie Universelle* (Paris, 1876–94))

Controlling state: Austria
Situation: Danube river port, left bank, at the junction with river Cerna, upstream of the Iron Gate. Town now in Romania and rebuilt on higher ground following engineering works on the Danube.
Sources: Quin (1834), Marmont (1834), Paget (1835), Pardoe (1836), Minet (1837), Elliott (1837), Best (1839), Monson (1839), Olin (1840), Andersen (1841), Snow (1841), Fisk (1842), Pfeiffer (1842), Paton (1843), Wilson (1843), Marmier (c. 1844)

Comments:

Sometimes confused with New Orsova, a nearby Turkish fortress town on an island (since submerged). Pfeiffer thought Old Orsova (the first Austrian town on the upstream route) 'has rather a pretty effect', and Paget agreed it was a 'pretty little village'.[246] Elliott and Olin, respectively, found it 'beautifully' and 'romantically' positioned.[247] The town was famous for its market, described by Quin, Paget, Monson, Snow and Marmier, conducted under quarantine rules between Austrians, Hungarians, Wallachians and Serbs.[248] The lazaretto at Schuppanneck (also called Xupaneck), one and a half miles from town, had mixed reviews. Marmont called it a '*beau lazaret*' with nothing spared to give it the importance it deserved.[249] Paget knew 'few places where it [i.e. quarantine] would be more tolerable than at Orsova'.[250] Julia Pardoe, however, found conditions bad, describing 'cells' built around a central square garden, each approached by an entrance court paved with stone, and she criticized the fixed menu and sour wine from the government-controlled restaurant.[251] Minet thought the accommodation could be better.[252] But Best praised a 'magnificent establishment' perfectly arranged, with the restaurant supplying food and furnishings at advertised prices.[253] The lazaretto was described fully by Andersen, who was unimpressed by the layout of 'chambers' around a central garden while the food was gross.[254] Fisk reckoned travellers 'who have endured a Turkish quarantine will be little disposed to complain of an Austrian one'.[255] Quarantine still functioned for Paton, but Marmier found the system in decline.[256] Wilson was detained for only a few hours, and this 'durance vile' was less tiresome than the customs formalities.[257]

OTRANTO

QS number: 34

Controlling state: Naples
Situation: Italian Adriatic seaport
Sources: Casanova (1744), Evers (1779), Morritt (1795), Bramsen (1814), Laurent (1819)

Comments:

Permanent quarantine was maintained against the Ionian Islands (as at Ancona), but Casanova found he could land at the *parlatorio* of the health office.[258] There was no lazaretto, but Evers had the use of a house one mile from town with subsequent upgrade 'to a larger house, which had a tolerable garden, and was pleasantly situated close to the sea'.[259] The lazaretto was at Barletta (q.v.), to which many travellers continued their voyage as the sailing time from Otranto counted towards the period of quarantine.[260] In the nineteenth century, quarantine at Otranto was possible in 'a miserable convent' outside town which, although a large building, had no furniture, no fireplaces and only small unglazed windows.[261]

PIRAEUS

QS number: 35

Controlling state: Greece
Situation: Seaport for Athens
Sources: Strickland (c. 1835), Napier (c.1840), Murray (1840), Wilkinson (1843), Carlisle (1854), Murray (1854), Tobin (1854), Twain (1867)

Comments:

The first lazaretto, according to Strickland, was a fishing boat moored in the harbour. Quarantine could be endured in a cabin, 5 feet × 4 feet 3 inches and approached by a trap door from the deck, or passed with equal misery in the fish hold.[262] Napier stayed on board HMS *Beacon*.[263] Murray noted in 1840: 'there is now a spacious building on the shores of the Piraeus, recently constructed behind the Custom-house, for the special purposes of a Lazaretto'.[264] He called the rooms 'tolerable', but provisions were quite expensive. Wilkinson criticized 'the exorbitant charge of 5 shillings a day' for accommodation.[265] Carlisle underwent a 24-hour 'foolish quarantine' on board his ship.[266] Catherine Tobin's 24-hour detention was at 'airy apartments in the Lazzaretto' with furniture from a hotel and a decent dinner.[267] By 1854, Murray considered Piraeus among the four best lazarettos in the Mediterranean.[268] In subsequent cholera epidemics, quarantine was considerably lengthened, causing Twain notoriously to jump ship to visit the Acropolis.[269]

PORT MAHON

QS number: 36

N° 141. — PORT-MAHON.

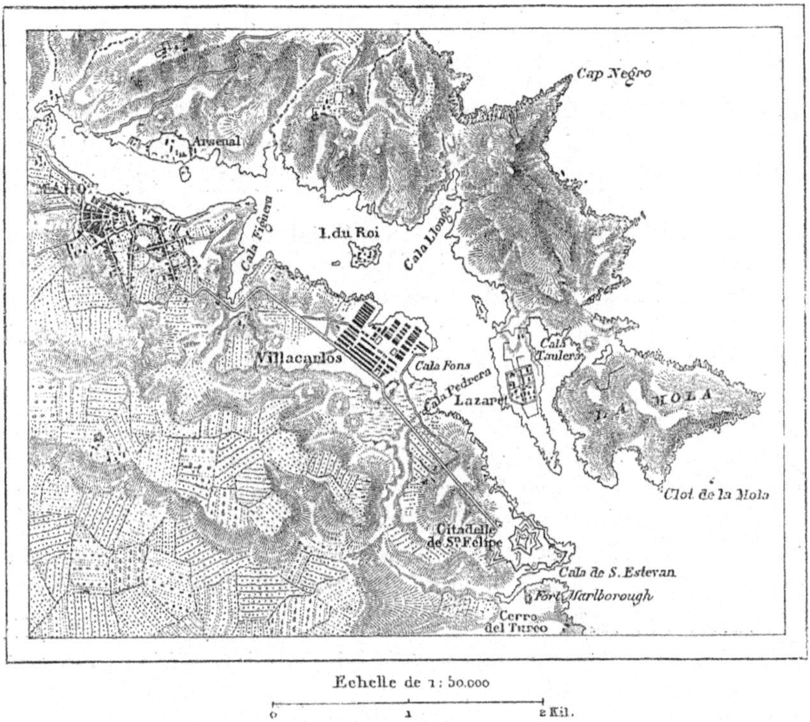

Illustration 36 The large harbour of Port Mahon, Minorca, showing the 'Lazaret' on a peninsula. The little island shown above the peninsula was the original 'Quarantine Island'.

Source: Reclus, E., *Nouvelle Géographie Universelle* (Paris, 1876–94)

Controlling state: Britain from 1708; France from 1756; Britain from 1763; Spain from 1782; Britain from 1798; Spain from 1802

Situation: Minorca, Balearic Islands

Sources: Comelin (1720), Woodruff (1828), Rockwell (c. 1835), Montague (1848), Panzac (1986), Booker (2007)

Comments:

The British struggled to find funds (and the cooperation of locals) to build a lazaretto on Quarantine Island in Mahon Harbour.[270] When materials were finally assembled, the island fell to the French, who abandoned the project.

When the British resumed control, the lazaretto was eventually built between 1767 and 1770, but it was cheap and flimsy. The Spanish, in 1793, decided to build a 'proper' lazaretto on the peninsula to the east of the island, but the British again struggled to complete it. The Spanish abandoned routine detention on Quarantine Island in 1817, despite having improved the lazaretto, and quarantine thereafter was normally limited to the peninsula, where the building could serve also as a barracks. In times of pandemic, however, especially of cholera, Quarantine Island served as an isolation hospital.

Minorca was never on a regular route for returning travellers, but it became a stopover for American merchantmen and men-of-war and occasionally for returnees from Barbary. Comelin was one of the latter and landed at Quarantine Island before the lazaretto was built.[271] Woodruff stayed on his ship, as did most Americans, but visited the peninsular lazaretto from curiosity.[272] His fellow countryman, Rockwell, arriving at a time of epidemic, found an American warship detained for cholera, with 700 of her 900 crewmen on Quarantine Island.[273] Montague was banned from landing at all as the master of his ship was suffering from varioloid, a mild form of smallpox, and was taken to the lazaretto. In his absence, the vessel was fumigated and all aboard received a vaccine in the ship's 'dispensary'. Outgoing letters were 'smoked' on Quarantine Island, which also yielded 'a very peculiar grass' that Montague dried between the pages of a book. The old lazaretto building was 'a cold, chilly, cheerless looking place . . . surrounded by high stone walls, with big doors painted red, with window-shutters half glass and half wood'.[274] The peninsular lazaretto closed in the 1930s and became a hotel.[275]

PRUTH, RIVER

QS number: 37

Controlling state: Russia

Situation: The boundary between Moldavia and Bessarabia, now the boundary between Romania and Moldova

Sources: Wittman (1802), Elliott (c.1837), Demidoff (1837), Terry (1847), Bush (1860s)

Comments:

There were several quarantine stations in the Pruth (now Prut) valley, all very bad and established largely for political reasons to prevent western influence in southern Russia. Consequently, there was the unusual misfortune of quarantine in a journey from west to east. For Wittman, however, the quarantine was conventional in that he was travelling northwestwards into Austrian-held territory at Chernowich (modern Chernivtsi in Ukraine). He found the station 'pleasantly situated at the side of the river Prut'.[276] Elliott, on the other hand, travelling eastwards into Russia at Liova (now Leova), had a nightmarish experience. He was delayed in a wretched hamlet on the Moldavian side, watching the sluggish Pruth, 'and the eye could not penetrate the dense vapor that arose from its surface'. All was squalor, mud and misery. Eventually, he crossed the river with others 'in a canoe formed of an excavated tree' and stumbled into the Russian quarantine consisting of several 'little detached buildings, surrounded by a wooden palisade forming a square of about a hundred and fifty yards'. They were sent back across the river by the bureaucratic commissary, returning the next day to face an absurd and bewildering interrogation complicated by insuperable problems of language and religion. Elliott's room, which he shared with others, was eleven feet square and seven feet high with a brick floor: 'it contained a stove, a small deal table, a wooden stool, and two frames of bedsteads, supplied with narrow planks which did not nearly meet one another'. Outside, there was 'a small enclosure, six yards square, in which a soldier . . . remained night and day'.[277]

The experience of Demidoff was slightly better. He crossed the Pruth upstream from Liova at Skoulani (now Sculeni). The Russian quarantine station occupied

> 'a large space, on a low and damp tract, the level of which barely rises above that of the waters of the Pruth. . . . At the least rise in the waters, the quarantine is inundated. . . . Nine small buildings of clay, covered with cane, compose this lazaretto. . . . The houses consist only of one floor, which is damp and sandy; they are divided into two or three small apartments, and are under the inspection of a keeper, an old soldier.'[278]

Terry noted a quarantine station at Reni, just north of the confluence of the Pruth and the Danube, but was too annoyed about its *raison d'être* (obstructing 'the light of knowledge') to comment on conditions.[279] Also at Reni, Eliza Bush noted 'a good stone house built for a quarantine here'.[280]

RAGUSA

QS number: 38

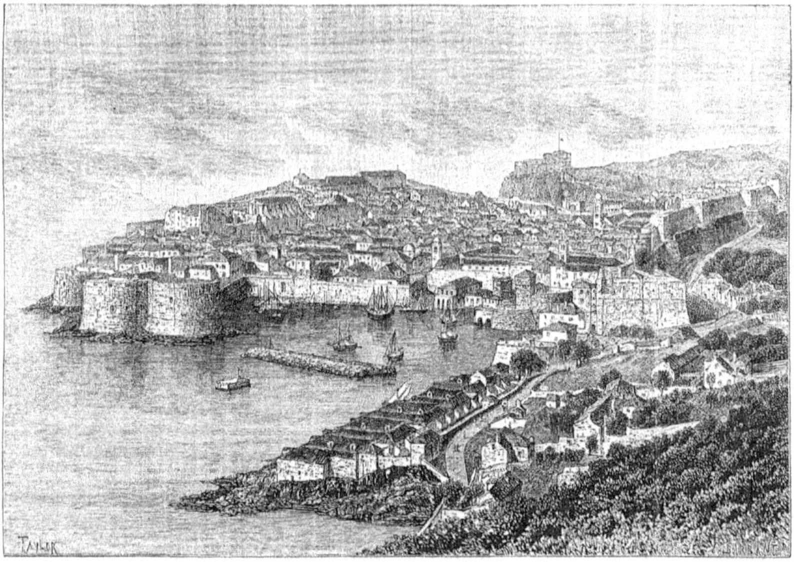

RAGUSE. — VUE PRISE DE PLOTCHÉ
Dessin de Taylor, d'après une photographie.

Illustration 37 Quarantine at Ragusa, the modern Dubrovnik, was in the range of buildings along the edge of the sea, to the right of the harbour mole.

Source: Reclus, E., *Nouvelle Géographie Universelle* (Paris, 1876–94)

Controlling state: Independent city under Venetian influence from the mid-fourteenth to early nineteenth century. Thereafter, briefly under French rule and then Austrian (Austro-Hungarian) until 1918, when it became part of Yugoslavia and was renamed Dubrovnik. In Croatia since 1991.
Situation: Eastern Adriatic seaport
Sources: Pouqueville (1798), Panzac (1986)

Comments:

An extremely old quarantine port (Panzac believes the system there could predate the one in Venice), which had no fewer than four lazarettos before the end of the seventeenth century.[281] The last one is still a feature of the approach to the inner harbour, notable for its windowless elevation towards the sea, but nonetheless picturesque. Pouqueville mentioned people who were quarantined there from Scutari before proceeding to Ancona,[282] but the irony is that this well-equipped port was virtually unused by western travellers. Its facilities were soon eclipsed by those at Venice, and as Venice itself lost out to Leghorn and Marseilles, so Ragusa was even more isolated from the arteries of travel.

RENI: *SEE UNDER* PRUTH, RIVER

ROTHENTHURN

QS number: 39

Controlling state: Germany, later Austria
Situation: Pass in Carpathian Mountains at frontier with Wallachia, on road to Hermannstadt (now Sibiu) in Transylvania. All now within Romania.
Sources: Hunter (1792), Jackson (1797), Clarke (1802), Lagarde (1811), Walsh (c. 1826), Frankland (1827)

Comments:

Also spelt Rothenturn (modern Rotenturm) and called Tour Rouge, named 'from a castle of that colour' about four miles past the quarantine station.[283] The remote pass, in the valley of the river Alt, was approached amid spectacular and beautiful scenery. This route was preferred to the Danube by some travellers as quarantine was allegedly one-third shorter.[284] Hunter, who claimed to have been 'almost starved', described the lazaretto as 'about a dozen white-washed houses' of one room devoid of movable furniture, each holding a bed of fixed, raised planks topped with prickly hay.[285] Jackson enjoyed 'plenty of the best provisions, wine, and fruits', but he had powerful letters of introduction.[286] Clarke, apparently with no letters, also had no complaints, having 'slept in the Director's house'.[287]

Lagarde stated that the lazaretto was properly built, comprising large warehouses for merchandise and '*plusieurs petites maisons*' for travellers who were segregated according to the probability of contagion. There was also a church, a barracks and a priest's house – in short, '*une ville en miniature*'.[288] Walsh summed up the site as 'about twenty houses, with a chapel, and a little inn, forming a village embosomed in high wooded hills'. Six of the houses were for personnel, including the director, while those for quarantine detainees were only wooden huts, plastered and whitewashed, each 'in a little dirty yard' surrounded by a nine-foot fence. Walsh thought nothing could 'be more revolting than the manner in which the traveller is received, or more dismal and disgusting than the place in which he is shut up'. He endured a nightmare detention with filthy conditions, foul smells and disgusting food.[289] Frankland, travelling south and therefore in pratique, was given 'a ham and three loaves of bread' by the director's wife, who took pity on his lack of resources.[290]

SANTA MAURA

QS number: 40

Controlling state: Venetian Republic to 1797; France to 1799; part of the Septinsular Republic to 1807; France to 1814; Britain to 1864; Greece thereafter
Situation: One of the Greek Ionian Islands, now Lefkada
Sources: Hennen (1830), Minet (1835), Lear (1848), Spencer (1850)

Comments:

Hennen described quarantine on the island as strict but 'on a small and mean scale'. He did not mention a lazaretto but claimed that the 'small sandy islet, about two miles to the northward of the north-eastern extremity of the isthmus, is fitted up for the purposes of quarantine; it is called the island of Saint Nicholas'.[291] Minet encountered an acquaintance who had been 20 days in the 'lazaretto', where three of his companions allegedly contracted plague.[292] Lear endured a nine-day detention, but his journal ended without comment on the place or the conditions.[293] Spencer, on the other hand, had plenty to talk about: his experience was horrific. He was conducted to his quarantine room,

> 'something in the form of a horse's crib, built of unplaned boards, and plastered inside and out with pitch; it measured exactly five feet by seven, about six feet in height, without chair or seat of any kind whatever; and this was one of the abodes for the higher class of travellers.'

Others made do 'with a shed similar to a market stall'. Spencer roasted in searing heat, plagued by mosquitoes and scorpions from a nearby swamp. After five days and nights in this 'baker's oven', he was predictably ill, shivering and shaking, crazed by thirst and fever, and reduced 'to a skeleton'.[294] After release he owed his life to the care of British soldiers who were protecting their country's interests on the island, while the control of quarantine remained in local hands.

SEMLIN

QS number: 41

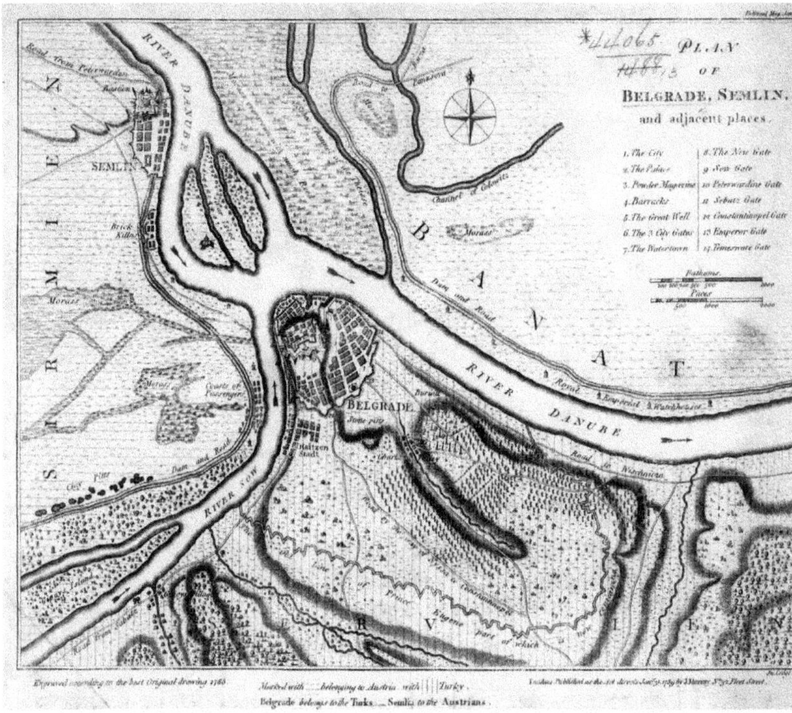

Illustration 38 The site of the quarantine river port of Semlin, the last Austrian town on the right bank of the Danube before Turkish-held Belgrade.

Source: © The British Library Board, Maps 44065(13)

Controlling state: Austria

Situation: Danube river port, right bank, at junction with river Sava (or Save). Now in Serbia and called Zemun.

Sources: Lusignan (1786), Keppel (1829), Burgess (1834), Kinglake (1834), Hervé (c. 1834), Paget (1835), Gleig (1837), Elliott (c.1837), Monson (1839), Murray (1840), Paton (1843), Marmier (c. 1845), Simpson (1846), Pridham (1849)

Comments:

A fortified town of multi-ethnic inhabitants, the starting point for excursions under quarantine to Turkish-held Belgrade and the last place in Austria on the right bank of the Danube. Paget thought the town 'contains some tolerable streets in the interior, but the part near the Danube looks as

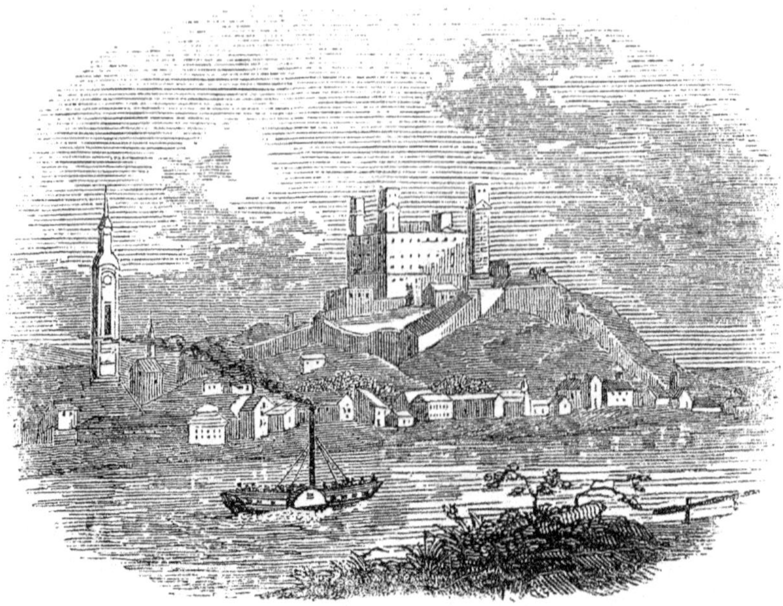

Illustration 39 A Danube steamer, typical of those taking travellers to Semlin, passes Presburg (now Bratislava) around 1835.

Source: Spencer, E., *Travels in Circassia, Krim Tartary, &c* . . . (London, 1837)

miserable as need be'.[295] Gleig agreed it was 'a poor, mean, deserted-looking town', while Monson scowled at the 'miserable looking village, surrounded by a wooden palisade'.[296] Paton called the lower town 'frightfully insalubrious, but the cemetery enjoys a high and airy situation. The people of the town die off with great rapidity, but, to compensate for this, the dead are said to be in a highly satisfactory state of preservation'.[297] Marmier was not inclined to such dry humour and dismissed the town as '*triste et misérable, sans industrie et sans commerce*'.[298] The lazaretto was called 'comfortable' by Murray, but food and bedding were supplied by a local inn 'at an exorbitant price'.[299] Keppel discovered that this inn was one mile away, to the detriment of the food it sent him. His quarters were

> 'truly miserable . . . a stone room, with two small windows, a brick floor, and a wooden platform . . . running round two sides. . . . This, and a stove, formed the only furniture I had the first night.'[300]

Burgess occupied a 'dwelling' of 100 feet × 60 feet, consisting of two bedrooms each 15 feet square, a kitchen between them, and a disproportionately large but 'convenient' passageway. He shared this space with three other travellers, a servant and a guardian. His courtyard was five yards × six yards. Burgess also noted that the lazaretto was 'set round with a rude pallisade [*sic*], except on the side where some dependencies afford additional comforts to the inmates'. He did not find the quarantine 'irksome' but was annoyed afterwards by 'harpies' in 'their taxing-den, called a Custom-house'.[301] Hervé 'had a very small house or cottage' with 'only one habitable room, a sort of loft above it, a kitchen, and a wash-house behind, with a little green plot of turf, on which we could stretch our legs'. He found the restaurateur sent over 'a good repast'.[302] Gleig described the lazaretto as 'a certain number of cells, with their respective yards or courts palisaded round' like cages in a zoo. There were also 'lodgings' for the guards, a detached house for 'the medical officers' and two churches, one Roman Catholic and the other Greek Orthodox.[303] Quarantine had evidently been discontinued by 1849 when Pridham reached Semlin from Bulgaria.[304] Panzac, who dates the lazaretto to as early as 1730, notes that the buildings were demolished in 1872 and the site made a public park.[305]

SMYRNA

QS number: 42

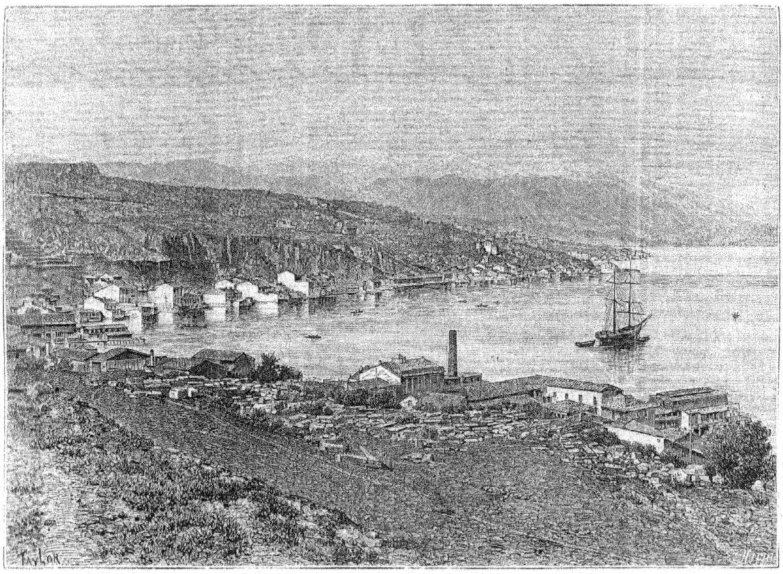

GOLFE DE SMYRNE. — VUE GÉNÉRALE DE KARA TACH ET DE GIOZ-TÉPÉ

Dessin de Taylor, d'après une photographie communiquée par M. Héron.

Illustration 40 The lazaretto at Smyrna was on the coast outside the city. The position would have been very similar to this.

Source: Reclus, E., *Nouvelle Géographie Universelle* (Paris, 1876–94)

Controlling state: Turkey (Ottoman Empire)
Situation: Aegean seaport, now Izmir
Sources: Olin (1840), Temple (1843), Wilson (1843), Gingras (1845), Gadsby (1847), Patterson (1850), Bryant (1853)

Comments:

Smyrna was the main port against which quarantine in the West was routinely enforced. It therefore came as a shock for travellers to be quarantined there themselves when Turkey adopted western ways. Olin and his party were especially upset, coming only from Syria and learning they 'were to be the first victims' of a 15-day detention. They managed to spend ten days on their steamer but were then escorted to 'some vile old house close to the sea shore, a mile or more below the city'. At least this was better than the 'foul lazaretto' to which his fellow non-western passengers had been sent immediately and where they 'suffered grievously . . . obliged to sleep upon the ground, many of them without covering, and half famished for want of food'.[306] Both Olin and Temple were supported by local missionary contacts; Temple was more philosophical about his delay but agreed that the lazaretto offered only 'bare walls'.[307] Wilson, by contrast, struck lucky. He was originally 'landed at the quarantine establishment, about a couple of miles from the town on the southern shore', but a fellow traveller gained permission to rent 'a cottage in a vineyard, for the accommodation of himself and friends, in which the Turks promised to allow them to go through their purgations'. Wilson was included in the party, and they passed their quarantine 'in the most agreeable manner'.[308]

Gingras called the lazaretto a virtual shack without furniture or amenities, but as it was too small to accommodate the six people in his party at once, he too was allowed to join an acquaintance in a rented house.[309] Perhaps luckily for Gadsby, his vessel was not even allowed to dock despite representations by the captain and physician to the health office.[310] Patterson, however, struck a positive note, reckoning that his place of confinement 'about a mile from Smyrna by the sea side' was 'rather better than the usual run of lazzarettos; but the intense heat renders the confinement irksome'.[311] Bryant wrote a letter from his 'chamber' in the lazaretto, which he described as a 'long, yellow building' near the shore, but curiously did not comment on conditions.[312]

SPALATRO
QS number: 43

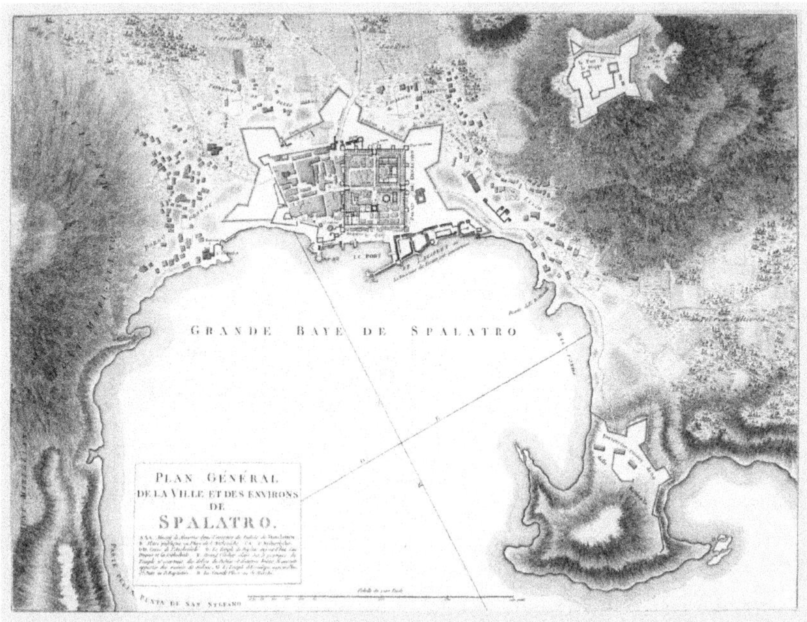

Illustration 41 This plan of Spalatro, around 1800, clearly marks 'Le Lazareht' to the east of the port.

Source: © The British Library Board, Maps 149.d.27

Controlling state: Dalmatia, usually under Venetian control
Situation: Adriatic seaport, now Split in Croatia
Sources: Mundy (1620), Spon and Wheler (1676)

Comments:

The town was also known as Spalato. A large lazaretto was built in the late sixteenth century by the Venetians but never widely used by westerners because, like the one at Ragusa, it was not on one of the routes the West normally adopted. Mundy arrived overland from Turkey in a prestigious group who had the building to themselves. They received 'beddinge, lynnen, Tables, Chaires and necessaries, but not soe to every one'.[313] Spon and Wheler noted that the lazaretto was regarded as a palace suitable for the ambassador travelling in their company and that they stayed there as well '*faute d'hôtellerie dans la Ville*'. The space for passengers consisted of three rectangles of different sizes. Their own room was the best of half a

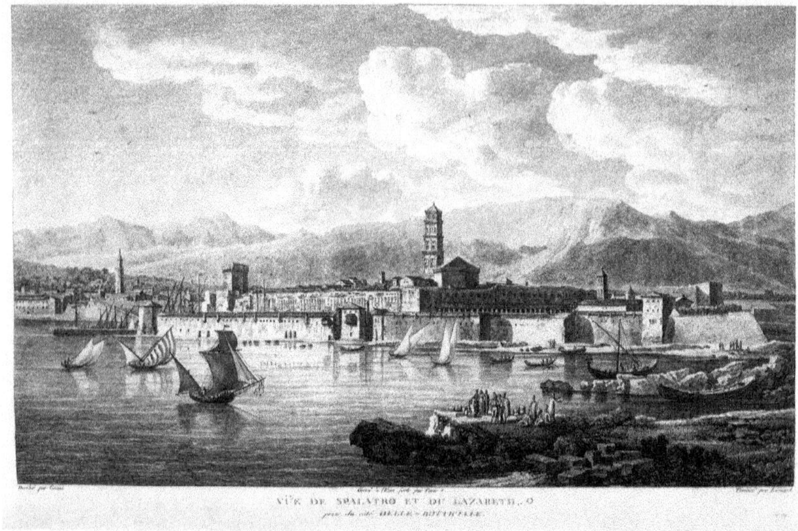

Illustration 42 The seaward elevation of the imposing Spalatro lazaretto.

Source: Cassas, L., *Voyage Pittoresque et Historique de l'Istria et de la Dalmatie* (Paris, 1802), via © The British Library Board, Maps 149.i.10

dozen in one rectangle, but they were unimpressed by the bare walls and nearly bitten to death by vermin.[314]

SYRA

QS number: 44

Controlling state: Greece
Situation: Island, now Syros, in the Cyclades, Aegean Sea
Sources: Auldjo (1833), Carne (1837), Knight (1838), Bowring (1838), Holroyd (1838), Usborne (c.1839), Murray (1840), Montefiore (1840), Beswick (1840), Londonderry (1840), Galton (1840), Scharf (1840), Stent (1842), Warburton (1843), Wilkinson (1843), Chenavard (1843), Tischendorff (1844), Watson (1845), Montauban (1845), Gadsby (1847), Bryant (1853), Carlisle (1853), Murray (1854), Hall (1855), Macaulay (1976), Slatter (1984), Panzac (1986)

Comments:

The most important by far of the several quarantine stations established in the 1830s by the newly autonomous Greek kingdom, following its rejection of the Ottoman yoke. Auldjo recognized this but appears to have stayed on board, perhaps unimpressed by conditions.[315] Certainly, the original building was awful. Carne reckoned that the

> 'most wretched of the houses of Syra would have been comfort compared to the interior of the lazaretto, which is a disgrace to Syra. . . . The walls rested on the native rock: the floors were of rock, only a boarding was raised in one part, four feet above the floor, and on this beds were laid: the rats ran in and out by dozens. . . . When it rained . . . the inmates were half drowned.'

And so his tirade continued.[316] Knight congratulated himself that he did not have to go there (having arrived in pratique from Nauplia), the more so as plague had allegedly appeared in the lazaretto that morning.[317]

Bowring claimed that 'the exactions' at Syra were 'monstrous, and where lately there was not even a water-proof roof to shelter an invalid'. He claimed also to have seen a man with rat-torn clothing and his body 'disfigured by multitudinous vermin'.[318] Holroyd, in response to his own questionnaire, learnt from the British consul at Syra that the lazaretto was 'in a very wretched condition' despite repairs, but that the Greek government was planning a new one, finances permitting, on the opposite side of the harbour.[319] Murray agreed that the lazaretto at Syra was 'abominable, and ought by all means to be avoided. It is composed of mere boxes of wood, which swarm with vermin'.[320] Usborne, as a casual visitor, breakfasted in the courtyard of the lazaretto with friends, who gave him such a good report of conditions that he resolved to pass his next quarantine there.[321] This is so out of step with earlier reports that it is difficult to deduce which lazaretto he visited.

The foundation stone of the new building was dated 9 April 1839,[322] so Montefiore was evidently one of the earliest residents. For the first night, more than ten of his party shared 'two miserably dark rooms'. But then he and his wife were given 'the apartments set aside for noblemen', which were 'very comfortable' although unfurnished initially, and with a pretty view.[323] The Beswicks, passing through in February 1840, thought the lazaretto looked 'a wretched place' and it was presumably the new one.[324] Lord Londonderry refused to do any quarantine at Syra, having been denied pratique for his yacht, and sailed on to Corfu 'setting the Greek authorities at defiance'.[325] He noted elsewhere in his diaries that the lazaretto at Syra was 'was cold comfortless, and abominable in all ways', but that was apparently hearsay.[326]

Galton had rooms which 'opened at the back into a cheerful covered balcony which looked on the sea', and he rather enjoyed his quarantine. He described the lazaretto as enclosing a large square, and it was in that 'little square before our row of houses' that Scharf wiled away moonlit evenings.[327] For Stent, however, the 'large airy lazaretto' recently built was a disappointment: 'it is advisable for the wretched incarcerated travellers to bring their own bedding and other comforts'.[328] Warburton, on the other hand, was satisfied with his apartment, although the 'prison looked dismal enough as the stormy evening set in, and the wind howled round the naked walls and desolate rocks of our dwelling'.[329] Wilkinson advised that the lazaretto 'is said to be pretty comfortable', which implies he had never been there.[330] Chenavard was definitely unimpressed, having to sleep on the stone floor of a cold cell because he arrived one rainy night without notice.[331] By contrast, those who arrived on a summer's day took everything in their stride: Tischendorff was bowled over by the beauty of the view and the breaking of the waves below his window.[332]

Watson took in the panorama from his ship, deciding to stay aboard, while Mrs Montauban thought the prospect of the lazaretto from the sea was 'neat'.[333] But tales of Syra's miserable past were slow to die, and even in 1847 Gadsby heard that 'the lazaretto was reputed to be one of the filthiest in the Mediterranean'.[334] For later travellers, such as Bryant, Carlisle and Hall, quarantine was too brief to incite caustic comment, but Murray, in 1854, described Syra as among the four best lazarettos in the Mediterranean, a radical change from the guidebook's view some 14 years earlier.[335] The building became disused after 1860 and served various uses (including a barracks and a prison) before partial demolition in the 1970s.[336]

SYRACUSE

QS number: 45

Controlling state: Sicily; Naples (Kingdom of the Two Sicilies) from 1816
Situation: Mediterranean seaport
Sources: Denon (1778), D'Irumberry (1791), Monson (1819), Wilson (1820), Sherer (1823)

Comments:

Denon landed 'at a wretched hovel, called the Health Office', from which he was conducted to a 'lazaretto' consisting of 'a hillock of ten paces square, without any shelter'. The authorities offered the following day 'to build a hut for us at our expense'. Denon declined as they 'had not come to Syracuse for the express purpose of building a lazaretto', and it was conceded that they could haul their boat ashore and live in it. He remarked that the lazarettos of Sicily were farmed and the farmers were only interested in profit.[337] It irritated both merchants and travellers (such as Wilson) that quarantine in Sicily was routinely imposed against Malta, although D'Irumberry escaped it at Syracuse by appealing to the governor.[338] Monson was not so lucky and was given 21 days. Having seen on the quayside some wooden sheds 'not unlike cow-houses' which passed for a lazaretto, he reacted as Denon had done by returning to his ship, where the crew 'erected an awning' to sit out the detention. The futility of Sicilian quarantine was brought home to him by the evenings he then passed with another Briton who arrived later, also from Malta. This man was in the lazaretto, but Monson was able to join him at will: 'one of the merriest evenings I ever passed, was the one before we left quarantine, when, *tous ensemble*, we drank the health of old England in that miserable shed under the walls of Syracuse'.[339] This same 'shed' had equally bad press from Sherer, who bemoaned his 'eleven days in a wretched wooden building, set apart for a lazaretto'.[340]

TREBIZOND

QS number: 46

Controlling state: Turkey
Situation: Black Sea port, now Trabzon
Sources: Perkins (1841), Wolff (1845), Sheil (1853)

Comments:

Perkins found the whole experience 'an amusing farce'. He and his wife had been given leave to pass their quarantine in a private house, but as it held other guests heading east, they stayed initially in their tent. Supervision of their quarantine 'was committed to our guardiano, who, instead of urging strictness in its observance, contrived various methods to help us through it as superficially as possible'.[341] Wolff was no more impressed: 'It is strange to hear of quarantine on land, and it is one of the most foolish things I ever heard of'. But he was treated well, allocated a room 'close by the ambassador of Bokhara'.[342] Lady Sheil, on the other hand, was slightly disgruntled:

> 'We are undergoing here the ordeal of a ten days' quarantine, to remind us, I suppose, that we are on the threshold of Europe. If we were more comfortably lodged, the repose after our harassing journey would be rather a luxury than otherwise.'[343]

TRIESTE

QS number: 47

N° 80. — TRIESTE.

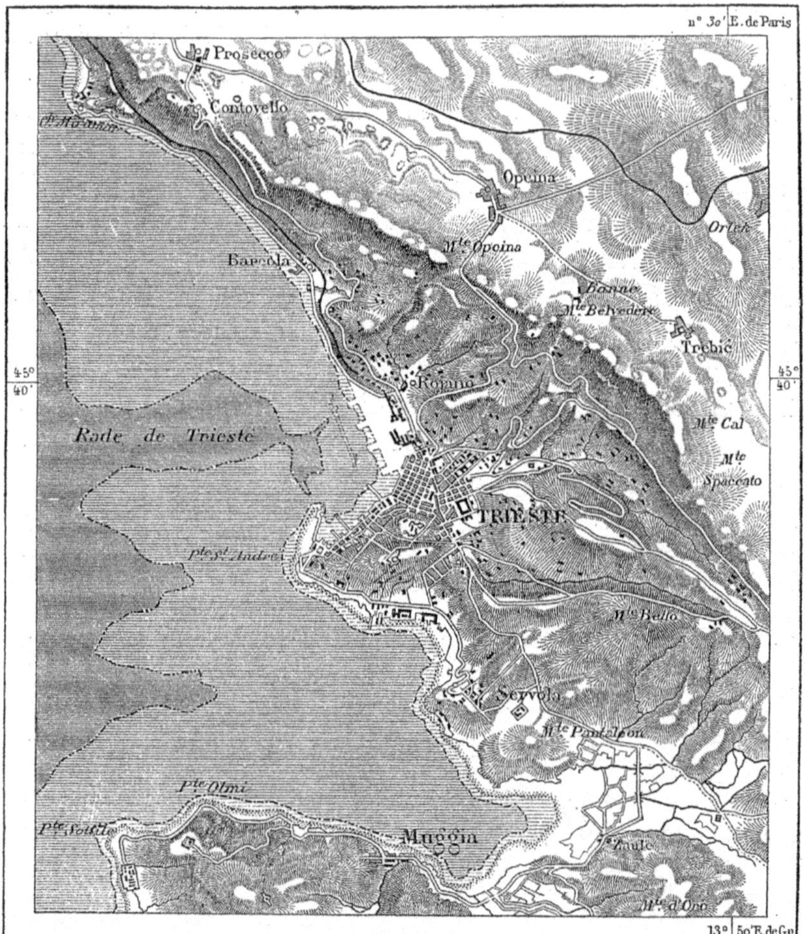

D'après l'Etat-Major Autrichien — Gravé par Erhard

Echelle de 1: 100.000

Kil. 0 1 2 3 4 5

Ligne donnant la profondeur d'environ 5 mètres.
Profondeurs de 10 mètres.
Profondeurs de 20 mètres

Illustration 43 The port of Muggia, at the bottom of the map, succeeded Trieste as a quarantine station.

Source: Reclus, E., *Nouvelle Géographie Universelle* (Paris, 1876–94)

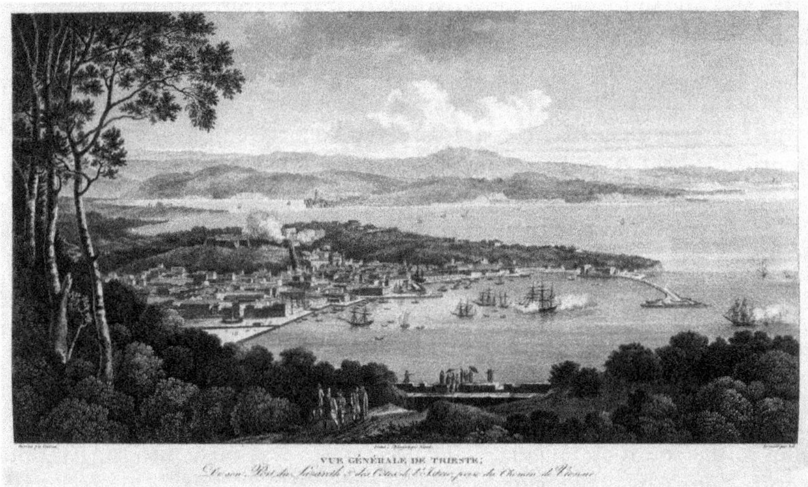

Illustration 44 Trieste port. The buildings at the shore end of the harbour mole, towards the right of the picture, formed the first lazaretto. A later and grander lazaretto was built to the north of the harbour – on this print the site is obscured by trees.

Source: Cassas, L., *Voyage Pittoresque et Historique de l'Istria et de la Dalmatie* (Paris, 1802), via © The British Library Board, Maps 149.i.10

Controlling state: Austria
Situation: Adriatic seaport, now in Italy
Sources: Howard (1785), Howel (1788), Biddle (1806), Turner (1817), Quin (1834), Usborne (c. 1838), Scharf (1840), Heywood (1845), Russell (1851), Panzac (1986)

Comments:

The city was a relatively late developer, slow to gain entry to the clique of major quarantine ports, but by the nineteenth century it had superseded many of its rivals. Usborne commended Trieste as having 'more the appearance of a great capital than seven-eighths of those so called', and Heywood agreed it was a 'wonderfully well-built town' with 'streets truly magnificent'.[344] As a quarantine station it was respected and efficient with a good reputation among diners. The first lazaretto (known later as the Old Lazaretto) was built south of the port in the 1720s.[345] This building was eclipsed (but not entirely superseded) from 1769 by the more spacious New Lazaretto erected on the north side of the harbour by the Empress Maria Theresa, within a massive double wall. It comprised its own large harbour and 32 apartments. Howard reproduced plans and noted that the rooms were 18½ feet × 15 feet, each with 'a neat bedstead, chair and table', although some apartments were less well furnished.[346] Biddle called the Old Lazaretto 'less uncomfortable than I expected. It is a large building with decent chambers & things can be procured to eat & drink'.[347] Turner recorded that the New Lazaretto offered 'a neat room without a chimney, or any other furniture than a table and three wooden benches . . . outside of my room is a small antechamber over the staircase, with a large chimney for cooking'.[348] Scharf called the New Lazaretto

> 'large and square with a great red tiled sloping roof and in appearance like a convent . . . [with] colonnades and galleries round an open space like an Italian inn. Every thing is very clean and white [and] each room is numbered. . . . There are many guardians but none appointed to particular persons.'[349]

The New Lazaretto was demolished in 1867 in favour of another one some miles to the south at Muggia.[350] That lazaretto was busy into the twentieth century before its conversion into a barracks.[351]

VENICE

QS number: 48

Controlling state: Venetian Republic
Situation: Adriatic seaport
Sources: Canaye (1573), Pindar (1602), Carleton (1610), Mundy (1620), D'Alquie (1665), Spon & Wheler (1676), Bruyn (1684), Dumont (1691), Casanova (1745), Doidge (1758), Howard (1785), Macgill (1806), Panzac (1986)

Comments:
Arguably the oldest quarantine port in the world, but its reputation diminished in step with the waning of Venetian power. From the eighteenth century, very few travellers from the Levant passed their quarantine there, and in the nineteenth century the facilities were totally eclipsed by those at Trieste. With decline in use came a lowering of standards, so that Howard (who described the system at Venice in great detail) declared 'there is such remissness and corruption . . . so as to render the quarantine almost useless'.[352] The Old Lazaretto was built in the early fifteenth century and the New Lazaretto about 50 years later. Both of these were situated on islands in the Venice Lagoon. In 1782 another island, Poveglia, was adopted for quarantine, and the facilities were enlarged and modernized in the nineteenth century.[353] Its tourist use, however, was minimal. Early travellers were unspecific as to where they passed their quarantine, if they suffered it at all. Canaye only mentioned being sent for two days '*au lazaret*', and Ambassador Pindar limited his account to the compulsory opening of presents.[354] Carleton, another envoy, was detained at Crema (on the Venetian

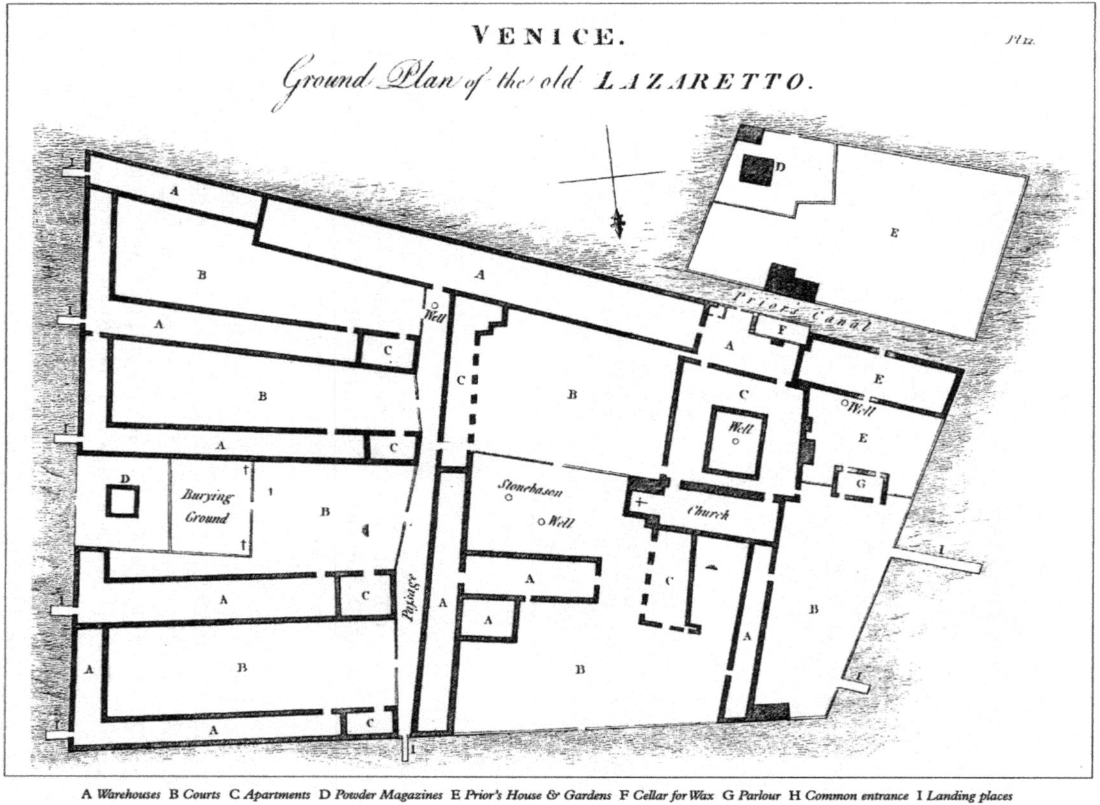

Illustration 45 Ground plan of the Old Lazaretto at Venice, surrounded by the waters of the Lagoon.

Source: Howard, J., *Principal Lazarettos in Europe* (London, 1791)

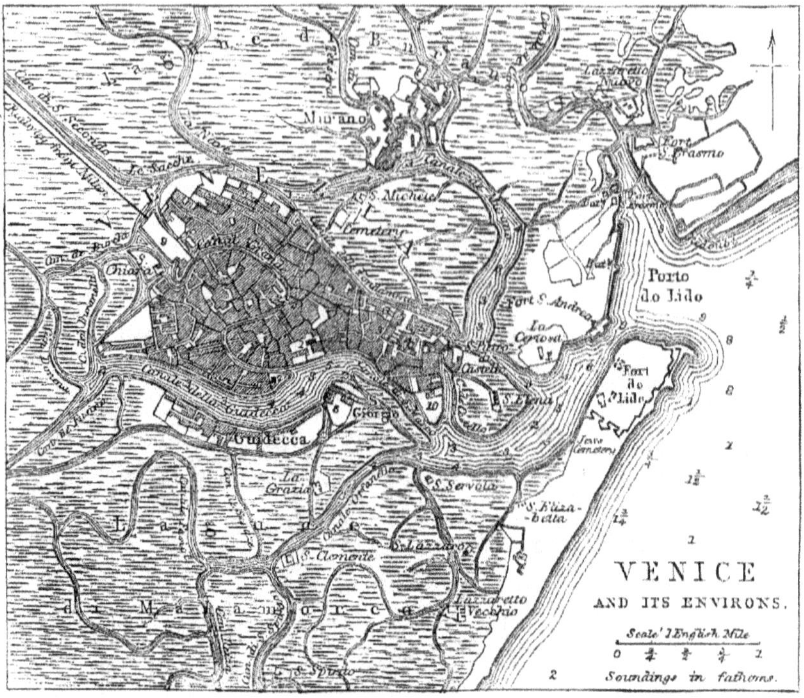

1 Church and Piazza di San Marco
2 Ponte di Rialto
3 Arsenal Vecchio
4 Arsenal Nuovo
5 Darsena Novissima Grande
6 Darsena della Galeazze
7 Dogana, and Church of Santa Maria della Salute
8 Church of San Giorgio Maggiore
9 Railway Station
10 Giardini Publici

Illustration 46 Venice in the context of its Lagoon. The Old Lazaretto ('Lazzaretto Vecchio') is shown at the bottom (south) of the map, while the New Lazaretto ('Lazzaretto Nuovo') is near the top, to the right (east).

Source: *Imperial Gazetteer* (London, Glasgow & Edinburgh, 1878)

frontier) as his journey was overland, while Mundy was excused any delay as he had been quarantined at Spalatro.[355] D'Alquié disembarked at the Old Lazaretto, but the restrictions were hardly severe as he was visited by '*une bonne partie de la principale Noblesse de Venise*'.[356] Spon and Wheler were admitted to immediate pratique for the same reason as Mundy.[357]

Bruyn expatiated on quarantine theory without being too precise as to which lazaretto he was in: he mentioned only that the 'House of health is a Building standing in the Water Incompassed with a Wall' and contained 'several publick Apartments'.[358] Dumont, however, was specific. He described the Old Lazaretto as being one mile from the city (Howard called it two), while the New Lazaretto, where he was detained, was five miles away. It was a two-storey building, 300 paces long,

> 'divided by high Walls into six Apartments, each of which has a particular Gate that leads into a Square Court, where there is a Well, but the

Water is so bad, that we never use any but what is brought from *Venice*. Every Apartment contains Twenty Chambers, Ten above, and as many below, separated like Cells, with a Chimney in each.'[359]

Casanova managed to spend his 11 days of quarantine on board his ship; Doidge went to a lazaretto but gave no details.[360]

The brief description of the sites and facilities described by Macgill would almost suggest he had never seen them.[361] In fact, no one was half as forthcoming about conditions as Howard. He was towed in a small boat 'to the new lazaretto', where he found 'a very dirty room, full of vermin, and without table, chair, or bed'. As this lazaretto was 'chiefly assigned to Turks and soldiers', he applied successfully for transfer to the old one where he hoped conditions might be better. He did indeed have a larger apartment with an upper and a lower room, but it 'was no less disagreeable and offensive than the former'. Within a few days he was moved again, this time to a four-room apartment where the view was pleasant 'but the rooms were without furniture, very dirty, and no less offensive than the sick wards of the worst hospital'. Howard paid to have the walls lime-washed, which restored his health and his appetite.[362] Panzac notes that both lazarettos are now in ruins.[363]

ZANTE

QS number: 49

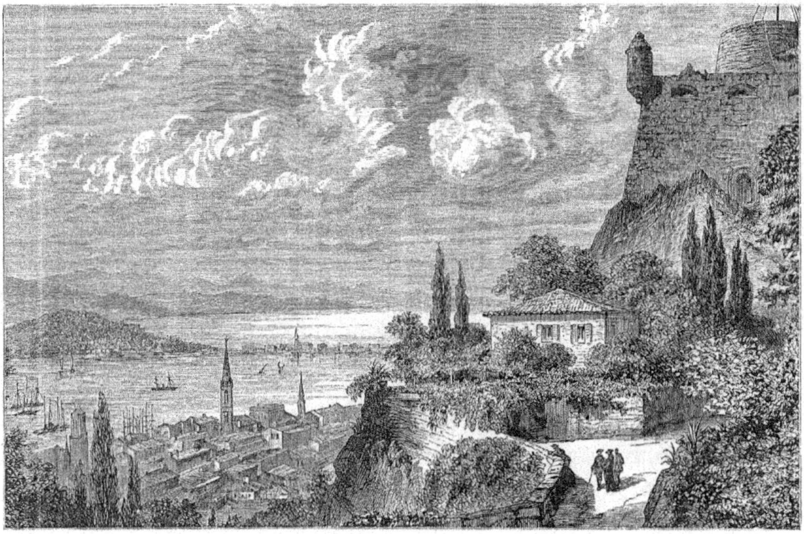

Illustration 47 A glimpse of shipping in the quarantine port of Zante.

Source: Hanson, C., *The Land of Greece Described and Illustrated* (London, 1886)

Controlling state: Venetian Republic; France from 1797; part of the Septinsular Republic from 1799; France from 1807; Britain from 1814; Greece from 1864

Situation: One of the Greek Ionian Islands, now Zakynthos

Sources: Dallam (1599), Sandys (1610), Carré (1674), Lucas (1703), Chandler (1766), Evers (1779), Howard (1785), Grasset (c.1791), Morritt (1795), Winterton (c. 1800), Turner (1813), Woods (1818), Allen (1819), Carne (1821), Trant (1829), Auldjo (1833), Minet (1835), Murray (1840)

Comments:

The lazaretto existed by 1599, the year when it was visited by Dallam who called it 'a prison'.[364] Sandys thought it more in 'the nature of a Pest-house'.[365] Lucas found only four walls, nothing to sleep on but a stone floor and nothing to eat at first but very black biscuits. Indeed, he claimed that he and the small child who accompanied him might well have perished there as the room was open to the sky with no possible shelter; his experiences are among the most harrowing ever recorded in quarantine history.[366] Chandler found conditions better: 'The lazaretto is by the sea-side, at a distance from the town. We were lodged over our servants and baggage in a chamber without any furniture, the walls white-washed'.[367] But at least they had a roof. Evers was told that the lazaretto was 'unhealthy' and not fit for a gentleman, so the British consul found him 'a very good house' near the health office.[368] Howard distinguished between the old and new lazarettos, but the latter was restricted to peasants returning from Greece after working on the harvest. The old lazaretto, by his day, had evidently improved, and Howard thought the layout afforded 'some good ideas for the construction of a house of correction'. He noted a covered gateway, with rooms either side and above for guards and officials, leading to an inner court of 130 feet × 35 feet. 'The doors of the other courts (three on each side) open into this. On one side they are chiefly designed for passengers, and in each there are four rooms, one of which having a fire-place is called the kitchen'. Each court had its own well and there were religious buildings nearby, including a convent.[369]

Grasset explained that passengers from ships at anchor, but only in passing, could come ashore to rest in a '*logement*', not the lazaretto, near the health office.[370] Under French rule, conditions apparently worsened, as Turner mentioned 'wretched accommodations' in the lazaretto where he caught a violent fever.[371] The British reintroduced a kind of segregation: Allen was relieved that the health officer 'would not let us go into the common Lazaretto, but sent for the keys of an old convent just behind it, which has also a garden, and had the rooms swept out for us'.[372] Carne had no such favours but was locked up in the lazaretto, which he detested.

> 'The apartment [which he shared with two Greeks] was about twelve feet square, with a stone floor, and two large open window places: frames

and glass might have been once there, but they had utterly disappeared; and the large door-way also had no door.'

But at least it was warm weather, the food was acceptable and the wine was good.[373] Trant was even more enthusiastic, 'delighted to enter the Lazaretto' after her hardships and to find the luxury of a bed.[374] Despite these positive comments, Murray's assessment comes as a surprise after the horrors of earlier years: 'Quarantine may be performed on Zante; the Lazaretto is the best, and the situation the healthiest of any of the [Ionian] islands'.[375]

Notes

Notes to follow referring to works in the bibliography are described minimally by the surname of the author. This name is followed by (a) date of publication (given to avoid ambiguity, typically when two authors share the same name); (b) volume number, if applicable, in lower-case Roman numerals; and (c) the page number(s). In a few cases those numbers will be in Roman when the reference is to introductory material in the work cited.

1 Trant (1830, 93).
2 Murray (1840, 16).
3 Pfeiffer (1851, 266).
4 Poujoulat (1840, ii, 436–7).
5 Walpole (1851, i, 253–4).
6 Wittman (1803, 420); Bramsen (1820, i, 184); Sherer (1825, 197).
7 D'Estourmel (1844, ii, 145).
8 Macbrair (1839, 118).
9 Scott (1837, i, 44–5).
10 Marmont (1837, iii, 124–6).
11 Bowring (1838, 12).
12 Robinson (1841, iii, 449).
13 Pfeiffer (1852, 216).
14 Beamont (1856, i, 56–7).
15 Maxwell (1882, 83).
16 For a full description of the site, see Panzac (1986, 154–5).
17 Olivier (1807, vi, 514–15).
18 Alcock (1831, 223).
19 Mure (1842, ii, 307).
20 British Library, Add. MS. 36448, ii, 3 July 1840.
21 Pridham (1851, 237–8).
22 Macintosh (1854, ii, 71).
23 Wilbraham (1839, 74–5).
24 Morritt (1914, 253).
25 Hughes (1820, ii, 363).
26 Laurent (1821, 258).
27 Grellet (1860, ii, 44).
28 Cambridge University Library, MSS. Dept., Add MS., 7633/1/86.
29 *British Parliamentary Papers* (1842, lxi, 614).
30 Bowring (1838, 13).
31 Millard (1843, 341).

32 Warburton (1845, ii, 55–6).
33 Nerval (1851, i, 314).
34 Kelly (1844, 53–4).
35 Galton (1908, 101–2).
36 Taylor (1855, 19).
37 Ibid., 20.
38 Andersen (1846, iii, 141). He called the town Widdin.
39 Skene (1853, i, 271–2).
40 Burton (1838, 268–9).
41 Ibid., 271.
42 Elliott (1838, i, 185).
43 Panzac (1986, 157).
44 Pococke (1745, ii, 179).
45 Grasset (1800, iii, 51).
46 Booker (2007, 410); Panzac (1986, 157).
47 Tafur (1926, 138).
48 Bowring (1838, 15); Best (1842, 236).
49 Slade (1840, 214–15).
50 Perkins (1843, 486).
51 Davy (1842, ii, 359).
52 Stent (1843, ii, 223).
53 Fisk (1844, 417).
54 Warburton (1845, ii, 364).
55 Ibid.
56 Heywood (1919, 44, 53).
57 Vigier (1886, 17).
58 Howard (1791, 10).
59 Olivier (1807, vi, 488); Dodwell (1819, i, 41).
60 Alcock (1831, 223); Best (1842, 3).
61 Vane (1844, 166).
62 Lear (1852, 415); Denison (1849, 192); Murray (1854, 16).
63 The plan is reproduced in Panzac (1986, 158).
64 Scott (1837, ii, 250–51), from which all references under Crete are taken.
65 Somerset Record Office, DD/SH/44/8.
66 Lumsden (1822, 180–1).
67 Ibid., 181.
68 Lyall (1825, ii, 190).
69 Ibid.
70 Ibid., 191.
71 Ibid.
72 Malherbe (1846, ii, 314–24), from which all references under El Arish are taken.
73 Best (1842, 297).
74 Pfeiffer (1852, 34–5).
75 Marmier (1846, i, 306).
76 Carlisle (1854, 38).
77 Spencer (1838, ii, 198).
78 Vane (1842, i, 151–2).
79 Marmier (1846, i, 306–7).
80 Boucher de Perthes (1855, ii, 394).
81 Ibid., 396.
82 Stent (1843, ii, 12).
83 Tischendorff (1847, 127).
84 Ibid., 128.

85 Spencer (1850, 245).
86 Neale (1852, i, 13).
87 Ibid.
88 Bryant (1869, 163).
89 Tobin (1855, 137–9).
90 Thomson (1859, ii, 334, 337).
91 Slade (1854, 540).
92 Panzac (1986, 167–9). Other plates are at the back of Howard (1791), who mentions the lazaretto (p. 7) but gives no description.
93 Labat (1730, ii, 58).
94 Sainte-Maure (1724, 198).
95 Rousseau (n.d., 273–4).
96 Howard (1791, 5–7).
97 Macbrair (1839, 23).
98 Panzac (1986, 163).
99 Bisani (1793, 203).
100 Brooke (1831, ii, 146).
101 Newman (c. 1961–2006, iii, 143–6).
102 Castlereagh (1847, ii, 302–3).
103 Hutton (1847, ii, 317).
104 Montague (1849, 328).
105 Baxter (1852, i, 124).
106 Brassey (1880, 207).
107 Maxwell (1882, 9).
108 Elliott (1838, i, 178–81).
109 Spencer (1851, ii, 410–11).
110 Perkins (1843, 123–4).
111 Gadsby (1880, 457).
112 Monk (1851, ii, 135).
113 Ibid., 140.
114 Minet (1958, 246).
115 Murray (1840, 16).
116 Measor (1844, 177).
117 Borrer (1845, 397–8).
118 Howard (1791, 7).
119 Mundy (1907, i, 16–17).
120 Fermanel (1664, 458–60).
121 Thévenot (1664, 566–8).
122 Carré (1947–8, iii, 931).
123 Tournefort (1718, ii, 398).
124 Labat (1730, ii, 126).
125 Saumery (1732–5, iv, 135–52).
126 Grosley (1769, ii, 329–30).
127 Prutky (1991, 499).
128 Ives (1773, 393–400).
129 La Lande (1790, ii, 420–1).
130 Binos (1798, ii, 355).
131 Daschkaw (1840, i, 239–41).
132 Rooke (1783, 124).
133 Tully (1819, i, 208).
134 Sutherland (1790, 260–1); Granville (1916, i, 81).
135 Macgill (1808, ii, 184).
136 Semple (1808, ii, 23–4).

137 Dodwell (1819, ii, 466–7).
138 Trethewey (2002, 132).
139 Matthews (1820, 33).
140 Birmingham City Archives, Galton MS 3101/C/E/S/17/30; 3101/C/E/2/1/2.
141 Sinclair (1829, 296).
142 Buckingham and Chandos (1862, ii, 309); Valery (1839, 412–13).
143 Asmar (1844, ii, 260).
144 Minet (1958, 404).
145 Knight (1839, 317).
146 Fulchiron (1843–58, i, 5).
147 Panzac (1986, 173–6).
148 Sandwich (1799, 4).
149 Parbury (1841, 276).
150 Browne (1867, 305–14).
151 Booker (2007, 327–8).
152 Teonge (1927, 59).
153 Dumont (1705, 119).
154 Howard (1791, 8).
155 D'Irumberry (1799, 251); Byron (1973–82, ii, 44).
156 Cazenove (1813, 234).
157 Woods (1828, ii, 307).
158 Sherer (1825, 214).
159 Lushington (1829, 200): 'a just complaint may be made of the unnecessary privation of exercise'.
160 Montefiore (1836, 257).
161 MacGill (1839, 86).
162 Lushington (1829, 199).
163 Auldjo (1835, 239).
164 Scott (1900, v, 370).
165 Newman (1891, 332; c. 1961–2006, 188–9).
166 Frankland (1829, ii, 198).
167 Wilkinson (1843, i, 67; 1847, xxiii).
168 Waring (1843, 53).
169 Marchebeus (1839, 218–19).
170 Salle (1840, ii, 268).
171 Kinnear (1841, 307).
172 Damer (1841, ii, 254–5).
173 Beswick (1997, 34); Vane (1844, 194).
174 Griffith (1845, i, 78).
175 Malherbe (1846, 388).
176 Murray (1840, x).
177 Booker (2007, 523–4); Snow (1842, 76).
178 Stent (1843, i, 118).
179 Wilkinson (1843, i, 55).
180 Hervey (1846, ii, 61–6); Thackeray (1846, 61).
181 Griffith (1845, i, 80); Montauban (1846, 13).
182 Bevan (1849, 163).
183 Young (1848, 442).
184 Wilkinson (1847, xxiii).
185 Bevan (1849, 164).
186 Smith (1850, 285).
187 Baxter (1850, 273).
188 Panzac (1986, 172).

189 Ibid., 180.
190 Ibid., 181.
191 Carré (1947–8, 941).
192 Daniel (1949, 83); Comelin et al. (1735, 128).
193 Plaisted (1757, 145–8).
194 Howard (1791, 4).
195 Grellet (1860, i, 112–13).
196 Trant (1925, 38).
197 Tets (1966, 145).
198 Damoiseau (1839, ii, 235).
199 Malcolm (1897, 403).
200 Starke (1828, 466).
201 Stendhal (1932, 394–5, 401–2).
202 Rockwell (1842, ii, 17).
203 Pardoe (1838, i, 115–26).
204 Demidoff (1855, ii, 317).
205 Romer (1843, i, 189–90).
206 Wilkinson (1843, i, 55).
207 Galton (1908, 108).
208 Montague (1849, 325).
209 Gasparin (1848, iii, 476–7).
210 Panzac (1986, 181).
211 Lucas (1731, ii, 456).
212 Labat (1730, v, 180).
213 Pococke (1745, ii, 199); Nugent (1749, iii, 366).
214 Howard (1791), end of book.
215 Sutherland (1790, 259).
216 Caroline (1821, 697).
217 Lumsden (1822, 173).
218 Howard (1791, 8).
219 Panzac (1986, 186).
220 Swan (1826, i, 35).
221 Buckingham and Chandos (1862, ii, 147–8).
222 Cooper (1838, 92).
223 Twain (1875, 308; 1958, 74).
224 Scott (1853, 758).
225 Grosvenor (1842, i, 198–9).
226 Minet (1958, 226).
227 Senior (1871, ii, 54–5).
228 Reuilly (1806, 265–6).
229 Macgill (1808, ii, 185, 196).
230 Pinkerton (1833, 123–4).
231 Moore (1833, 144).
232 Marmont (1837, i, 177–8).
233 Craven (1868, i, 309, 311).
234 Ros (1855).
235 Stephens (1839, i, 261–2).
236 Spencer (1837, i, 218).
237 Stuart (1854, 360–1).
238 Hommaire de Hell (1847, 4).
239 Knight (1839, 206, 318); Bowring (1838, 12).
240 Slade (1840, 309–13).
241 Jesse (1841, i, 58).

242 Terry (1848, 246–56).
243 Scott (1854, 339).
244 Brooks (1854, 29).
245 M'Culloch (1882, 969).
246 Pfeiffer (1852, 28); Paget (1839, ii, 125).
247 Elliott (1838, i, 131); Olin (1843, ii, 475).
248 Quin (1835, i, 121); Paget (1839, ii, 125); Monson (1840, 145–6); Snow (1842, 32); Marmier (1846, i, 261–2).
249 Marmont (1837, i, 112–13).
250 Paget (1839, ii, 126).
251 Pardoe (1854, 331, 334).
252 Minet (1958, 426).
253 Best (1842, 322).
254 Andersen (1846, 169).
255 Fisk (1844, 442).
256 Paton (1845, 39); Marmier (1846, i, 261).
257 Wilson (1847, ii, 434).
258 Casanova (1958–60, i, 488).
259 Evers (1784, 150–1).
260 Morritt (1914, 253, 256); Laurent (1821, 256).
261 Bramsen (1820, ii, 124).
262 Strickland (1858, cxlii).
263 Napier (1842, ii, 358).
264 Murray (1840, 16).
265 Wilkinson (1843, i, 67–8).
266 Carlisle (1854, 314).
267 Tobin (1855, 241).
268 Murray (1854, 16).
269 Twain (1875, 340–53).
270 A synopsis of quarantine arrangements on Minorca is given in Booker (2007, 130–50).
271 Comelin et al. (1735, 122).
272 Woodruff (1831, 205–8).
273 Rockwell (1842, i, 31).
274 Montague (1849, 77–84).
275 Panzac (1986, 177–8).
276 Wittman (1803, 476).
277 Elliott (1838, i, 216–28).
278 Demidoff (1855, i, 232–3).
279 Terry (1848, 285).
280 Bush (1867, 287).
281 Panzac (1986, 160).
282 Pouqueville (1821, 453).
283 Walsh (1829, 301).
284 Jackson (1799, 264–5).
285 Hunter (1798, ii, 207–13).
286 Jackson (1799, 263–4).
287 Clarke (1818, viii, 282).
288 Lagarde (1824, 356).
289 Walsh (1829, 301–8).
290 Frankland (1829, i, 17).
291 Hennen (1830, 377–8).
292 Minet (1958, 253).

293 Lear (1852, 330).
294 Spencer (1851, ii, 212–15).
295 Paget (1839, ii, 90).
296 Gleig (1839, iii, 273); Monson (1840, 130).
297 Paton (1845, 42).
298 Marmier (1846, i, 213).
299 Murray (1840, 217–18).
300 Keppel (1831, i, 461).
301 Burgess (1835, ii, 289–90).
302 Hervé (1837, ii, 323–4).
303 Gleig (1839, iii, 277).
304 Pridham (1851, 188–9).
305 Panzac (1986, 201).
306 Olin (1843, ii, 468–70).
307 Temple (1855, 334–5).
308 Wilson (1847, ii, 422).
309 Gingras (1847, ii, 392–4).
310 Gadsby (1880, 93–4).
311 Patterson (1852, 338).
312 Bryant (1869, 186).
313 Mundy (1907, i, 87).
314 Spon and Wheler (1679, ii, 22–3).
315 Auldjo (1835, 204–5).
316 Carne (1836, ii, 37); cf. Slatter (1984, 76).
317 Knight (1839, 49–51).
318 Bowring (1838, 13).
319 Holroyd (1839, 45).
320 Murray (1840, 16) (acknowledging Bowring).
321 Usborne (1840, 83).
322 Macauley (1976, 17–18) transcribes the wording (in English) of the marble entrance plaque.
323 Montefiore (1890, i, 263).
324 Beswick (1997, 33).
325 Vane (1844, 163–4).
326 Vane (1842, ii, 37).
327 Galton (1908, 53); British Library, Add. MS. 36488; Slatter (1984, 75).
328 Stent (1843, i, 118), where the word Syra is misprinted as 'Syria'.
329 Warburton (1845, ii, 387).
330 Wilkinson (1843, i, 61).
331 Chenavard (1849, 157–8).
332 Tischendorff (1847, 282).
333 Watson (1853, 63–4); Montauban (1846, 17).
334 Gadsby (1880, 132).
335 Murray (1854, 16).
336 Panzac (1986, 192).
337 Denon (1789, 305–6).
338 Wilson (1824, 390–1); D'Irumberry (1799, 265).
339 Monson (1820, 185, 189–90).
340 Sherer (1825, 227).
341 Perkins (1843, 483).
342 Wolff (1848, 398).
343 Sheil (1856, 297).
344 Usborne (1840, 15); Heywood (1919, 68).

345 Panzac (1986, 195).
346 Howard (1791, 23).
347 Biddle (1993, 207).
348 Watson (1820, iii, 326).
349 British Library, Add. MS. 36488.
350 Panzac (1986, 196).
351 Ibid., 197.
352 Howard (1791, 22).
353 Panzac (1986, 199).
354 Canaye (1897, 208); Sanderson (1931, 222).
355 *Calendar of State Papers Venetian* (1905, xii, 1610–13; xxiv, 69); Mundy (1907, 89–90).
356 D'Alquié (1670–71, part 2, 127).
357 Spon and Wheler (1679, ii, 284).
358 Bruyn (1702, 285–6).
359 Dumont (1705, 349).
360 Casanova (1958–60, i, 533); Ives (1773, 397–9): Henry Doidge was a friend and correspondent.
361 Macgill (1808, ii, 180–1).
362 Howard (1791, 11).
363 Panzac (1986, 199).
364 Dallam (1893, 89).
365 Purchas (1905, 92).
366 Lucas (1731, ii, 435–44).
367 Chandler (1817, ii, 335–6).
368 Evers (1784, 132).
369 Howard (1791, 9–10).
370 Grasset (1800, iii, 189).
371 Turner (1820, i, 100).
372 Allen (1846, ii, 119).
373 Carne (1830, ii, 319).
374 Trant (1830, 344).
375 Murray (1840, 13).

Bibliography

Primary sources: manuscript

Birmingham City Archives: MS 3101 (Galton Papers)
British Library: Add. MS. 36488, 3 vols (Scharf diaries)
Cambridge University Library: Add. MS. 7633/1/86 (Kinglake Papers)
National Archives: PC 2 as far as 2/213 (Privy Council Papers
National Archives of Malta: C1–2 (Quarantine Office letter-books)
Somerset Record Office: DD/SH/44/8 (Strachey Papers)
University College London: Galton Papers 66
The Woburn Abbey Collection: 3/21/3 and 4/27/5 (6th Duke of Bedford)

Primary sources: printed

Abu, Taleb Khan, *Travels of Mirza Abu Taleb Khan in Asia, Africa, and Europe, During the Years 1799, 1800, 1801, 1802, and 1803 . . .*, Stewart, Charles (trans.), 3 vols (London, 1814)

Alcock, T., *Travels in Russia, Persia, Turkey, and Greece, in 1828–9* (described as 'not published', London, 1831)

Allen, W., *Life of William Allen with Selections from His Correspondence*, 3 vols (London, 1846)

Ampère, J.J., *Voyage en Egypte et en Nubie* (Paris, 1868)

Andersen, H.C., *A Poet's Bazaar: From the Danish of Hans Christian Andersen . . . by Charles Beckwith*, 3 vols (London, 1846)

Angas, G.F., *A Ramble in Malta and Sicily, in the Autumn of 1841* (London, 1842)

Anon, *Narration of Voyage* (In Library of American School of Classical Studies, Athens, n.d.)

Asmar, M.T., *Memoirs of a Babylonian Princess . . .*, 2 vols (London, 1844), reprinted in facsimile in Elibron Classics Series by Adamant Media Corporation (2003)

Auldjo, J., *Journal of a Visit to Constantinople, and Some of the Greek Islands, in the Spring and Summer of 1833* (London, 1835)

Baxter, W.E., *Impressions of Central and Southern Europe . . .* (London, 1850)

Baxter, W.E., *The Tagus and the Tiber; or, Notes of Travel in Portugal, Spain, and Italy, in 1850–1*, 2 vols (London, 1852)

Beamont, W., *A Diary of a Journey to the East in the Autumn of 1854*, 2 vols (London, 1856)

Beauvau, H. de, *Relation iournaliere du voyage du Levant faict & descript par Haut et puissant Seigneur Henry de Beauvau Baron du dict lieu . . .* (Nancy, 1619)

Beldam, J., *Recollections of Scenes and Institutions in Italy and the East*, 2 vols (London, 1851)

Best, Capt. J.J., *Excursions in Albania; Comprising a Description of the Wild Boar, Deer, and Woodcock Shooting in That Country; and from Thence to Thessalonica and Constantinople, and Up the Danube to Pest* (London, 1842)

Beswick, M. & Beswick, T., *Chronicles of a Journey 1839–1840: The Diaries of Mary & Tom Beswick of Gristhorpe of Their Travels to: Paris – Malta – Egypt – Naples – Rome – Florence – Lyon Paris and London*, Clegg, K. (ed.) (Filey, 1997)

Bevan, S., *Sand and Canvas: A Narrative of Adventures in Egypt, with a Sojourn Among the Artists in Rome* (London, 1849)

Biddle, N., *Nicholas Biddle in Greece: The Journals and Letters of 1806*, McNeal, R.A. (ed.) (University of Pennsylvania, Philadelphia, 1993)

Binos, L'Abbé de, *Voyage par l'Italie, en Egypte, au Mont-Liban et en Palestine, fait en 1777 et années suivantes . . .* , 2 vols (Paris, 1798)

Bisani, A., *A Picturesque Tour Through Part of Europe, Asia and Africa: . . . with Plates After Designs by James Stuart . . . Written by an Italian Gentleman* (London, 1793)

Borrer, D., *A Journey from Naples to Jerusalem, by Way of Athens, Egypt, and the Peninsula of Sinai . . .* (London, 1845)

Boucher de Perthes, J., *Voyage à Constantinople . . . En Mai, Juin, Juillet at Août 1853*, 2 vols (Paris, 1855)

Bowring, J., *Observations on the Oriental Plague and on Quarantines, as a Means of Arresting Its Progress . . .* (Edinburgh, 1838)

Bramsen, J., *Travels in Egypt, Syria, Cyprus, The Morea, Greece, Italy, &c. &c . . .*, 2nd ed., 2 vols (London, 1820)

Brassey, A., *Sunshine and Storm in the East, or Cruises to Cyprus and Constantinople* (London, 1880)

British Parliamentary Papers (London, 1842)

Brooke, Sir Arthur de Capell, Bart., *Sketches in Spain and Morocco*, 2 vols (London, 1831)

Brooks, C.W. Shirley, *The Russians of the South* (London, 1854)

Browne, J. Ross, *An American Family in Germany* (New York, 1867)

Bruyn, K.P. de, *A Voyage to the Levant: Or, Travels in the Principal Parts of Asia Minor, the Islands of Scio, Rhodes, Cyprus, &c . . .* (London, 1702)

Bryant, W.C., *Letters from the East* (London, 1869)

Brydone, P., *A Tour Through Sicily and Malta in a Series of Letters to William Beckford, Esq. of Somerly in Suffolk*, 2 vols (London, 1790)

Buckingham, J.S., *Autobiography of James Silk Buckingham; Including His Voyages, Travels, Adventures, Speculations, Successes and Failures . . .* , 2 vols (London, 1855)

Buckingham, J.S. & Chandos, K.G., *The Private Diary of Richard, Duke of Buckingham & Chandos, KG*, 3 vols (London, 1862)

Burgess, Revd R., *Greece and the Levant; or, Diary of a Summer's Excursion in 1834: With Epistolary Supplements*, 2 vols (London, 1835)

Burton, Revd N., *Narrative of a Voyage from Liverpool to Alexandria; Touching at the Island of Malta, and from Thence to Beirout in Syria; with a Journey to Jerusalem, Voyage from Jaffa to Cyprus and Constantinople, and a Pedestrian Journey from Constantinople, Through Turkey, Wallachia, Hungary, and Prussia, to the Town of Hamburgh, in the Years 1836–37* (Dublin, 1838)

Bush, E.C., *My Pilgrimage to Eastern Shrines* (London, 1867)

Bussolin, G., *Delle istituzioni di sanità marittima nel bacino del Mediterraneo* (Trieste, 1881)

Byron, Lord, *The Poetical Works of Lord Byron: A New Edition . . .*, 6 vols (London, 1855)

Byron, Lord, *'Famous in My Time': Byron's Letters and Journals*, Marchand, L.A. (ed.), 12 vols (John Murray, London, 1973–82)

Calendar of State Papers Venetian, 38 vols (London 1864–1947)

Calvert, F., *A Tour to the East in the Years 1763 and 1764: With Remarks on the City of Constantinople and the Turks . . . (6th Baron Baltimore)* (London, 1767)

Canaye, P. du Fresne, *Le Voyage du Levant de Phillipe du Fresne-Canaye (1573) publié et annoté par M.H. Hauser . . .* (Paris, 1897)

Carlisle, Earl of, *Diary in Turkish and Greek Waters* (London, 1854)

Carmichael, *see* Montauban, Mrs. E., *A Year and a Day in the East; or, Wanderings Over Land and Sea* (London, 1846)

Carne, J., *Letters from the East: Written During a Recent Tour Through Turkey, Egypt, Arabia, the Holy Land, Syria and Greece*, 3rd ed., 2 vols (London, 1830)

Carne, J., *Syria, the Holy Land, Asia Minor, &c. Illustrated in a Series of Views Drawn from Nature by W.H. Bartlett, William Purser, &c . . .*, 2 vols in one (London, Paris and America, 1836)

Caroline, Queen, *Voyages and Travels of Her Majesty, Caroline Queen of Great Britain . . .* (London, 1821)

Carré, Abbé, *The Travels of the Abbé Carré in India and the Near East 1672 to 1674 . . .*, 3 vols, Series II (Hakluyt Society, London 1947–8)

Casanova, J., *The Memoirs of Jacques Casanova de Seingalt: The First Complete and Unabridged English Translation by Arthur Machen*, 6 vols (G. P. Putnam's Sons, New York and London, 1958–60)

Cassas, L.F., *Voyage Pittoresque et Historique de L'Istria et de la Dalmatie, redigé . . . par Joseph Lavallée* (Paris, 1802)

Castlereagh, Viscount, *A Journey to Damascus Through Egypt, Nubia, Arabia Petraea, Palestine, and Syria*, 2 vols in one (London, 1847)

Cazenove, H., *A Narrative in Two Parts: Written in 1812* (London, 1813)

Chandler, R., *Travels in Asia Minor, and Greece: Or, an Account of a Tour Made at the Expense of the Society of Dilettanti*, 3rd ed., 2 vols in one (London, 1817)

Chenavard, A.M., *Voyage en Grèce et dans le Levant fait en 1843–1844 . . .* (Lyon, 1849)

Clarke, E.D., *Travels in Various Countries of Europe Asia and Africa . . .*, 4th ed., 11 vols (London, 1816–24)

Comelin, F., *et al.*, *A Voyage to Barbary, for the Redemption of Captives; Performed (in 1720) by the Mathurin-Trinitarian Fathers, Fran. Comelin, Philemon de la Motte, and Jos. Bernard* (London, 1735)

Cook, T., *Dr W.H. Russell of London, Consul Lever of Trieste and Cook's Tourists: Letters to His Royal Highness the Prince of Wales . . .* (London, 1870)

Cooper, J. Fenimore, *A Residence in France; with an Excursion up the Rhine, and a Second Visit to Switzerland*, 2 vols (London, 1836)

Cooper, J. Fenimore, *Excursions in Italy* (Paris, 1838)

Cornille, H., *Souvenirs D'Orient*, 2nd ed. (Paris, 1836)
Craven, Augustus [Craven, P.M.A.A.], *A Sister's Story . . . Translated from the French by Emily Bowles*, 3 vols (London, 1868)
D'Alquié, F.S., *Les Memoires du Voyage de Monsieur le Marquis de Ville au Levant . . .*, 3 parts (Amsterdam, 1670–71)
Dallam, T., *Early Voyages and Travels in the Levant. 1.- The Diary of Master Thomas Dallam, 1599–1600.11. Extracts from the Diaries of Dr. John Covell, 1670-1679 . . . Edited . . . by J. Theodore Bent . . .*, 87 vols (Hakluyt Society, London, 1893)
Damer, Hon. Mrs. G.L., *Diary of a Tour in Greece, Turkey, Egypt, and the Holy Land*, 2 vols (London, 1841)
Damoiseau, L., *Voyage en Syrie et dans le Désert*, 2 vols in one (Brussels, 1839)
Daniel, W., *The Red Sea and Adjacent Countries at the Close of the Seventeenth Century as Described by Joseph Pitts William Daniel and Charles Jacques Poncet Edited by Sir William Foster . . .*, Series II, 100 vols (Hakluyt Society, London, 1949)
Daschkaw Bradford, W. (ed.), *Memoirs of the Princess Daschkaw, Lady of Honour to Catherine II Empress of all the Russias: Written by Herself . . .*, 2 vols (London, 1840)
Davy, J., *Notes and Observations on the Ionian Islands and Malta: With Some Remarks on Constantinople and Turkey, and on the System of Quarantine as at Present Conducted*, 2 vols (London, 1842)
Demidoff, A., *Travels in Southern Russia, and the Crimea; Through Hungary, Wallachia, & Moldavia, During the Year 1837*, 2 vols (London, 1855)
Denison, Lord Albert, *Wanderings in Search of Health* (London, 1849)
Denon, D.V., *Travels in Sicily and Malta: Translated from the French of M. De Non, Gentleman in Ordinary to the King of France, and Member of the Royal Academy of Painting and Sculpture* (London, 1789)
D'Estourmel, J., *Journal d'un Voyage en Orient . . .*, 2 vols (Paris, 1844)
D'Irumberry, C.M., Comte de Salaberry, *Voyage à Constantinople, en Italie, et aux îles de l'Archipel, par l'Allemagne et la Hongrie* (Paris, 1799)
Dodwell, E., *A Classical and Topographical Tour Through Greece, During the Years 1801, 1805, and 1806*, 2 vols (London, 1819)
Dreux, R.P. Robert de, *Voyage en Turquie et en Grèce du R.P. Robert de Dreux aumonier de l'Ambassadeur de France (1665–1669) publié et annoté par Hubert Pernot . . .* (Les Belles Lettres, Paris, 1925)
Dumont, J., Baron de Carlscroon, *A New Voyage to the Levant: containing an Account of the Most Remarkable Curiosities in Germany, France, Italy, Malta, and Turkey . . .*, 4th ed. (London, 1705)
Dunlop, M. & Dunlop, R., *Two Sisters, The Timely Retreat; or A Year in Bengal Before The Mutinies*, 2nd ed., 2 vols (London, 1858)
Elliott, C.B., *Travels in the Three Great Empires of Austria, Russia, and Turkey*, 2 vols (London, 1838)
Evers, S., *A Journal Kept on a Journey from Bassora to Bagdad; Over the Little Deset* [sic], *to Aleppo, Cyprus, Rhodes, Zante, Corfu; and Otranto, in Italy; in the Year 1779. By a Gentleman, Late an Officer in the Service of the Honourable East-India Company; Containing an Account of the Progress of Caravans Over the Desert of Arabia; Mode and Expences of Quarantine . . .* (Horsham, 1784)
Fane, H.E., *Five Years in India . . .*, 2 vols (London, 1842)

Fermanel, *Le Voyage D'Italie et Du Levant, de Messieurs Fermanel . . . Fauvel . . . Baudouin de Lavnay: et de Stochove . . .* (Rouen, 1664)

Field, J., *Correspondence of John Howard, the Philanthropist* (London, 1855)

Fisk, Revd G., *A Pastor's Memorial of Egypt, the Red Sea, the Wildernesses of Sin and Para, Mount Sinai, Jerusalem, and Other Principal Localities of the Holy Land, Visited in 1842 . . .*, 2nd ed. (London and Wolverhampton, 1844)

Fitzclarence, Lt-Colonel G. [Earl of Munster], *Journal of a Route Across India, Through Egypt, to England, in the Latter End of the Year 1817, and the Beginning of 1818* (London, 1819)

Fitzmaurice, Hon. W.E., *A Cruise to Egypt, Palestine, and Greece, During Five Months' Leave of Absence* (London, 1834)

Forbin, Comte de, *Travels in Egypt, Being a Continuation of the Travels in the Holy Land, in 1817–18* (London, 1819a)

Forbin, Comte de, *Voyage dans le Levant* (Paris, 1819b)

Formby, Revd H., *A Visit to the East; Comprising Germany and the Danube, Constantinople, Asia Minor, Egypt, and Idumea* (London, 1843)

Frankland, Capt. C.C., *Travels to and from Constantinople, in the Years 1827 and 1828 . . .*, 2 vols (London, 1829)

Frankland, Capt. C.C., *Narrative of a Visit to the Courts of Russia and Sweden, in the Years 1830 and 1831*, 2 vols (London, 1832)

Fraser, J.B., *A Winter's Journey . . . from Constantinople to Tehran; with Travels Through Various Parts of Persia, &c.*, 2 vols (London, 1838)

Freygang, W. von, *Letters from the Caucasus and Georgia; to Which Are Added, the Account of a Journey into Persia in 1812 . . .* (London, 1823)

Fulchiron, J.-C., *Voyage dans L'Italie Méridionale*, 2nd ed., 7 vols (Paris, 1843–58)

Gadsby, J., *My Wanderings: Being Travels in the East in 1846–47, 1850–51, 1852–53*, revised ed. (London, 1880)

Galton, F., *Memories of My Life* (London, 1908)

Gardiner, W., *Sights in Italy . . .* (London, n.d.)

Gasparin, Madame de, *Journal d'un Voyage au Levant par l'Auteur du Mariage au point de vue Chrétien*, 3 vols in one (Paris, 1848)

Gell, Sir W., *Narrative of a Journey in the Morea* (London, 1823)

Géramb, M.-J. de, *Pèlerinage à Jerusalem et au Mont-Sinaï en 1831, 1832 et 1833*, 3 vols (Paris, 1839)

Gingras, L., *L'Orient, ou Voyage en Egypte, en Arabie, en Terre-Sainte, en Turquie et en Grèce*, 2 vols (Quebec, 1847)

Giraudeau, J., *L'Italie, La Sicile, Malte, La Grèce, L'Archipel, Les Iles Ioniennes et La Turquie, Souvenirs de Voyage historiques et anecdotiques*, 2nd ed. (Paris, 1835)

Gleig, Revd G.R., *Germany, Bohemia, and Hungary, Visited in 1837*, 3 vols (London, 1839)

Granville, Countess C. (ed.), *Lord Granville Leveson Gower (First Earl Granville) Private Correspondence 1781 to 1821*, 2 vols (London, 1916)

Grasset de Saint-Sauveur, A., *Voyage historique, littéraire et pittoresque dans les isles et possessions, ci-devant vénitiennes du Levant*, 3 vols (Paris, 1800)

Grellet, S., *Memoirs of the Life and Gospel Labours of Stephen Grellet*, Seebohm, Benjamin (ed.), 2 vols (London, 1860)

Griffith, L.D., *A Journey, Across the Desert, from Ceylon to Marseilles: Comprising Sketches of Aden, the Red Sea, Lower Egypt, Malta, Sicily, and Italy*, 2 vols (London, 1845)

Grosley, P.J., *New Observations on Italy and its Inhabitants: Written in French by Two Swedish Gentlemen. Translated into English by Thomas Nugent . . .*, 2 vols (London, 1770)

Grosvenor, Lady E.M. [i.e. Marchioness of Westminster], *Narrative of a Yacht Voyage in the Mediterranean During the Years 1840–41*, 2 vols (London, 1842)

Gunn, J.A.W., *et al.* (eds.), *Benjamin Disraeli: Letters: 1815–1834* (Toronto and London, 1982)

Habeeb, Effendi Risk Allah, *The Thistle and the Cedar of Lebanon* (London, 1853)

Hall, H.B., *Sayah or, the Courier to the East* (London, 1856)

Hansard, T.C., *Hansard's Parliamentary Debates: Third Series* (London, 1842–3)

Hanson, C.H., *The Land of Greece Described and Illustrated* (London, 1886)

Haverty, M., *Wanderings in Spain in 1853* (London, 1844)

Hennen, J., *Sketches of the Medical Topography of the Mediterranean: Comprising an Account of Gibraltar, the Ionian Islands, and Malta* (London, 1830)

Hervé, F., *A Residence in Greece and Turkey; with Notes of the Journey Through Bulgaria, Servia, Hungary, and the Balkan*, 2 vols (London, 1837)

Hervey, A.H.A., *The Ocean & the Desert, by a Madras Officer*, 2 vols (London, 1846)

Heywood, R., *A Journey to the Levant in 1845* (Privately Printed, S.l., 1919)

Holroyd, A.T., *The Quarantine Laws, Their Abuses and Inconsistencies: A Letter Addressed to the Hon. Sir John Cam Hobhouse, Bart. M.P. President of the Board of Control, &c. &c. &c.* (London and Edinburgh, 1839)

Holthaus, P.D., *Wanderings of a Journeyman Tailor Through Europe and the East, During the Years 1824 to 1840*, Howitt, W. (trans.) (London, 1844)

Hommaire de Hell, X., *Travels in the Steppes of the Caspian Sea, the Crimea, the Caucasus, &c.* (London, 1847)

Howard, J., *An Account of the Principal Lazarettos in Europe . . .* (Warrington, 1789; London, 1791)

Howel, T., *A Journal of the Passage from India, by a Route Partly Unfrequented, Through Armenia and Natolia, or Asia Minor . . .* (London, 1788)

Hughes, Revd T. Smart, *Travels in Sicily Greece and Albania*, 2 vols (London, 1820)

Hunter, W., *Travels in the Year 1792 Through France, Turkey, and Hungary, to Vienna . . .*, 2 vols (London, 1798)

Hutton, R.N., *Five Years in the East*, 2 vols (London, 1847)

Inglis, H.D., *Spain in 1830*, 2 vols (London, 1831)

Irby, Hon. C.L. & Mangles, J., *Travels in Egypt and Nubia, Syria, and Asia Minor; During the Years 1817 & 1818* (London, 1823)

Ives, E., *A Voyage from England to India, in the Year MDCCLIV . . . Also, a Journey from Persia to England, by an Unusual Route . . .* (London, 1773)

Jackson, J., *Journey from India, Towards England, in the Year 1797; . . . and Through Romalia, Bulgaria, Wallachia, Transylvania, &c in Europe . . .* (London, 1799)

Jesse, Capt. W., *Notes of a Half-Pay in Search of Health: Or, Russia, Circassia, and the Crimea, in 1839–40*, 2 vols (London, 1841)

Johnes, M., *The Boy's Book of Modern Travel and Adventure* (London, 1859)

Kelly, W.K., *Syria and the Holy Land, Their Scenery and Their People . . .* (London, 1844)

Keppel, Capt. the Hon. G., *Personal Narrative of a Journey from India to England, by Bussorah, Bagdad, the Ruins of Babylon . . . in the Year 1824*, 2nd ed., 2 vols (London, 1827)

Keppel, Major the Hon. G., *Narrative of a Journey Across the Balcan, by the Two Passes of Selimno and Pravadi; also of a Visit to Azani . . . in the Years 1829–30*, 2 vols (London, 1831)

Kinglake, A.W., *Eothen, or Traces of Travel Brought Home from the East* (London, 1844)

Kinnear, J.G., *Cairo, Petra, and Damascus in 1839 . . .* (London, 1841)

Klaproth, J. von, *Travels in the Caucasus and Georgia, Performed in the Years 1807 and 1808 by Command of the Russian Government*, Shoberl, F (trans.) (London, 1814)

Knight, W., *Oriental Outlines or a Rambler's Recollections of a Tour in Turkey, Greece, & Tuscany in 1838* (London, 1839)

La Lande, M. de, *Voyage en Italie . . .*, 7 vols (Geneva, 1790)

Labat, P., *Voyages du P. Labat de L'Ordre des FF. Prescheurs, en Espagne et en Italie*, 6 vols (Paris, 1730)

Lagarde, Comte de, *Voyage de Moscou à Vienne, par Kiow, Odessa, Constantinople, Bucharest et Hermanstadt . . .* (Paris, 1824)

Laurent, P.E., *Recollections of a Classical Tour Through Various Parts of Greece, Turkey, and Italy, Made in the Years 1818 & 1819* (London, 1821)

Layard, Sir H., *Early Adventures in Persia, Susiana, and Babylonia . . .* , 2 vols (London, 1887)

Lear, E., *Journals of a Landscape Painter in Albania, Illyria, &c.*, 2nd ed. (London, 1852)

Lennep, Revd H. J. van, *Travels in Little-Known Parts of Asia Minor . . .* , 2 vols (London, 1870)

Letters from several Parts of Europe, and the East: Written in the Years 1750, &c . . ., 2 vols (Oxford, 1753)

Londonderry, *see* Vane, F.A., Londonderry, Marchioness of, *Narrative of a Visit to the Courts of Vienna, Constantinople, Athens, Naples, &c.* (London, 1844).

Lucas, P., *Voyage du Sieur Paul Lucas au Levant*, new ed., 2 vols (Paris, 1731)

Lumsden, Lt. T., *A Journey from Merut in India, to London, Through Arabia, Persia, Armenia, Georgia, Russia, Austria, Switzerland, and France, during the Years 1819 and 1820 . . .* (London and Edinburgh, 1822)

Lushington, C., *Narrative of a Journey from Calcutta to Europe by way of Egypt, in the Years 1827 and 1828* (London, 1829)

Lusignan, S., *A Series of Letters: Addressed to Sir William Fordyce, M.D. F.R.S . . .*, 2 vols (London, 1788)

Lyall, R., *Travels in Russia, the Krimea, the Caucasus, and Georgia*, 2 vols (London, 1825)

Macbrair, R. Maxwell, *Sketches of a Missionary's Travels in Egypt, Syria, Western Africa, &c, &c* (London, 1839)

Macgill, T., *Travels in Turkey, Italy, and Russia, During the Years 1803, 1804, 1805, & 1806: With an Account of some of the Greek Islands*, 2 vols (Edinburgh, 1808)

MacGill, T., *A Hand Book, or Guide, for Strangers Visiting Malta* (Malta, 1839)

Macintosh, Maj. General A.F., *A Military Tour in European Turkey, the Crimea, and on the Eastern Shores of the Black Sea . . .* , 2 vols (London, 1854)

Maclean, C., *An Excursion in France, and Other Parts of the Continent of Europe; from the Cessation of Hostilities in 1801, to the 13th of December 1803 . . .* (London, 1804)

Maclean, C., *Evils of Quarantine Laws, and Non-Existence of Pestilential Contagion* . . . (London, 1824)

Macleod, N., *Eastward* (London and New York, 1866)

M'Culloch, J.R., *A Dictionary . . . of Commerce and Commercial Navigation* (London, 1882)

Malcolm, A., *Letters of an Invalid from Italy, Malta, and the South of France* (50 copies only) (London, 1897)

Malherbe, R. de, *L'Orient 1718–1845 Histoire, Politique, Religion, Moeurs, Etc.*, 2 vols (Paris, 1846)

Marchebeus, *Voyage de Paris à Constantinople par bateau à Vapeur: Nouvel Itinéraire* . . . (Paris, 1839)

Marmier, X., *Du Rhin au Nil . . . Souvenirs de Voyages*, 2 vols (Paris, 1846)

Marmont, Viesse de, *Voyage du Maréchal Duc de Raguse en Hongrie, en Transylvanie, dans la Russe Méridionale, en Crimée, et sur les bords de la MerAzoff, à Constantinople, dans quelques parties de l'Asie-Mineure, en Syrie, en Palestine et en Egypte*, 5 vols (Paris, 1837)

Matthews, H., *The Diary of an Invalid Being the Journal of a Tour in Pursuit of Health in Portugal Italy Switzerland and France in the Years 1817, 1818 and 1819*, 2nd ed. (London, 1820)

Maxwell, General E.H., *Griffin Ahoy! A Yacht Cruise to the Levant, and Wanderings in Egypt, Syria, the Holy Land, Greece, and Italy, in 1881* (London, 1882)

Mead, R., *A Short Discourse Concerning Pestilential Contagion* . . . (London, 1720)

Measor, Revd H.P., *A Tour of Egypt, Arabia Petraea, and the Holy Land in the Years 1841–2* (London and Exeter, 1844)

Meryon, C.L., *Travels of Lady Hester Stanhope; Forming the Completion of Her Memoirs: Narrated by Her Physician*, 3 vols (London, 1846)

Millard, D., *A Journal of Travels in Egypt, Arabia Petrae, and the Holy Land, During 1841–2* (Rochester, 1843)

Minet, Susan (ed.), *Diary of James Minet 1807–1885: A Huguenot of the Fifth Generation* (Privately Printed, S.l., 1958)

Monk, C.J., *The Golden Horn; and Sketches in Asia Minor, Egypt, Syria, and the Hauraan*, 2 vols (London, 1851)

Monson, F.J. [Baron Monson], *Journal of a Tour in Germany, Through the Tyrol, Salzkammergut, the Danube, Hungary, &c. &c. &c. During the Months of August, September, and October, MDCCCXXXIX* ('not published', London, 1840)

Monson, W.J. [Baron Monson], *Extracts from a Journal* (London, 1820)

Montague, E.P. (ed.), *Narrative of the Late Expedition to the Dead Sea: From a Diary by One of the Party* (Philadelphia, 1849)

Montauban, E., *A Year and a Day in the East; or, Wanderings over Land and Sea* (London, 1846)

Montefiore, M., *Diaries of Sir Moses and Lady Montefiore*, Loewe, L. (ed.), 2 vols (London, 1890)

Montefiore, Mrs/Lady, *Private Journal of a Visit to Egypt and Palestine by Way of Italy and the Mediterranean* ('not published', London, 1836)

Moore, J., *A Journey from London to Odessa, with Notices of New Russia, etc.* (Paris, 1833)

Morritt, J.B.S., *The Letters of John B.S. Morritt of Rokeby Descriptive of Journeys in Europe in the Years 1794–1796*, Marindin, G.E. (ed.) (John Murray, London, 1914)

Moryson, F., *An Itinerary Containing His Ten Yeeres Travell Through the Twelve Dominions of Germany, Bohmerland, Sweitzerland, Netherland, Denmarke, Poland, Italy, Turky, France, England, Scotland & Ireland*, 4 vols (Glasgow, 1907–8)

Mundy, P., *The Travels of Peter Mundy in Europe and Asia, 1608–1667 . . .* , 5 vols, Second Series, no. 17 (Hakluyt Society, Cambridge, 1907)

Murdoch, J. Burn, *Notes and Remarks Made in Jersey, France, Italy, and the Mediterranean, in 1843 and 1844* (Edinburgh and London, 1846)

Mure, W., *Journal of a Tour in Greece and the Ionian Islands*, 2 vols (Edinburgh, London, 1842)

Murray, J., *A Hand-Book for Travellers in the Ionian Islands, Greece, Turkey, Asia Minor, and Constantinople . . .* (London, 1840)

Murray, J., *A Handbook for Travellers in Turkey . . .*, 3rd ed. (London, 1854)

Najaf Koolee Meerza, H.R.H., *Journal of a Residence in England, and of a Journey from and to Syria . . .*, Y. Kayat, Assaad (trans. with explanatory notes), 2 vols (Private Circulation, 1839)

Napier, Lt-Colonel, E., *Excursions Along the Shores of the Mediterranean*, 2 vols (London, 1842)

Napier, E. Major-General, *The Life and Correspondence of Admiral Sir Charles Napier, K.C.B., from Personal Recollections, Letters, and Official Documents*, 2 vols (London, 1862)

Neale, F.A., *Eight Years in Syria, Palestine, and Asia Minor, from 1842 to 1850*, 2 vols (London, 1852)

Nerval, Gérard de [Labrunie, Gérard], *Voyage en Orient*, 3rd ed., 2 vols (Paris, 1851)

Newman, J.H., and Mozley, A. (eds.), *Letters and Correspondence of John Henry Newman . . .* , 2 vols (London, 1891)

Newman, J.H., Ker, I. & Gornall, T. (eds.), *Letters and Diaries of John Henry Newman*, 31 vols (Clarendon Press, Oxford, c.1961–2006)

Nugent, T., *The Grand Tour: Containing an Exact Description of Most of the Cities, Towns, and Remarkable Places of Europe . . .* , 4 vols (London, 1749)

Olin, Rev. S., *Travels in Egypt, Arabia, Petraea, and the Holy Land*, 2 vols (New York, 1843)

Olivier, G.A., *Voyage dans l'Empire Othoman, L'Egypte et La Perse . . .* , 6 vols (Paris, 1807)

Paget, J., *Hungary and Transylvania; with Remarks on Their Condition, Social, Political, and Economical*, 2 vols (London, 1839)

Pallas, P.S., *Travels Through the Southern Provinces of the Russian Empire, in the Years 1793 and 1794. Translated from the German of P.S. Pallas, Counsellor of State to His Imperial Majesty of all the Russias . . .* , 2 vols (London, 1802–3)

Parbury, G., *Hand Book for India and Egypt, Comprising the Narrative of a Journey from Calcutta to England . . .* (London, 1841)

Pardoe, Miss, *The River and the Desart: Or, Recollections of the Rhône and the Chartreuse*, 2 vols (London, 1838)

Pardoe, Miss, *The City of the Sultan, and Domestic Manners of the Turks: With a Steam Voyage Up the Danube*, 4th ed. (London, 1854)

Parrot, Dr. F., *Journey to Ararat*, Cooley, W.D. (trans.) (London, 1845)

Paton, A.A., *Servia, the Youngest Member of the European family; or, a Residence in Belgrade, and Travels in the Highlands and Woodlands of the Interior, During the Years 1843 and 1844* (London, 1845)

Patterson, J.L., *Journal of a Tour in Egypt, Palestine, Syria, and Greece . . .* (London, 1852)

Perkins, Revd J., *A Residence of Eight Years in Persia, Among the Nestorian Christians; with Notices of the Muhammedans* (Andover, 1843)

Pfeiffer, I., *A Lady's Voyage Round the World: A Selected Translation from the German . . . by Mrs. Percy Sinnett* (London, 1851)

Pfeiffer, I., *Visit to the Holy Land, Egypt, and Italy . . . Translated from the German by H.W. Dulcken* (London, 1852)

Pinkerton, Revd R., *Extracts of Letters from the Rev. Robert Pinkerton, on His Late Tour in Russia, Poland, and Germany; to Promote the Object of the British and Foreign Bible Society* (London, 1817)

Pinkerton, Revd R., *Russia: Or, Miscellaneous Observations on the Past and Present State of That Country and Its Inhabitants . . .* (London, 1833)

Plaisted, B., *A Journal from Calcutta in Bengal, by Sea, to Busserah: From Thence Across the Great Desart [sic] to Aleppo: And From thence to Marseilles, and Through France, to England, in the Year, 1750 . . .* (London, 1757)

Pococke, R., *A Description of the East, and Some Other Countries*, 2 vols in 3 parts (London, 1745)

Poujoulat, B., *Voyage à Constantinople dans l'Asie Mineure, en Mésopotamie, à Palmyre, en Syrie, en Palestine et en Egypte*, 2 vols (Paris, 1840)

Pouqueville, F.C.H.L., *Voyage dans la Grèce . . .*, 5 vols (Paris, 1821)

Price, W., *Journal of Travels of the British Embassy to Persia; Through Armenia and Asia Minor, to Constantinople and Smyrna; . . . with the Voyage Back to England*, 2nd ed., 2 vols in one [vol. 1 title differs] (London, 1832)

Pridham, C., *Kossuth and Magyar Land, or, Personal Adventures During the War in Hungary* (London, 1851)

Prutky, R., *Prutky's Travels in Ethiopia and Other Countries Translated and Edited by J.H. Arrowsmith-Brown . . .*, Series II, 174 vols (Hakluyt Society, London, 1991)

Purchas, S., *Hakluytus Posthumus or Purchas His Pilgrimes . . .*, Extra Series, 8 vols (Hakluyt Society, Glasgow, 1905)

Quin, M.J., *A Steam Voyage Down the Danube: With Sketches of Hungary, Wallachia, Servia, and Turkey, &c*, 2nd ed., 2 vols (London, 1835)

Reclus, E., *Nouvelle Géographie Universelle . . .*, 19 vols (Paris, 1876–94)

Rees Van Tets, H.F., *Voyage D'Une Hollandaise en France en 1819 . . .* (Paris, 1966)

Rennie, Sir J., *Autobiography . . .* (London and New York, 1875)

Reuilly, J., *Voyage en Crimée et sur les Bords de la Mer Noire, pendant l'Année 1803 . . .* (Paris, 1806)

Roberts, E., *Notes of an Overland Journey Through France and Egypt to Bombay* (London, 1841)

Robinson, E., *Biblical Researches in Palestine, Mount Sinai and Arabia Petraea: A Journey of Travels in the Year 1838, by E. Robinson and E. Smith . . .*, 3 vols (London, 1841)

Rockwell, Revd C., *Sketches of Foreign Travel and Life at Sea; Including a Cruise on Board a Man-of-War, as also a Visit to Spain, Portugal, the South of France, Italy, Sicily, Malta, the Ionian Islands, Continental Greece, Liberia, and Brazil . . .*, 2 vols (Boston, 1842)

Rolt, R., *A New Dictionary of Trade and Commerce . . .* (London, 1756)

Romer, I.F., *The Rhone, the Darro, and the Guadalquivir; a Summer Ramble in 1842*, 2 vols (London, 1843)

Rooke, H., *Travels to the Coast of Arabia Felix; and from Thence by the Red-Sea and Egypt, to Europe . . .* (London, 1783)

Ros, Lord de, *Journal of a Tour in the Principalities, Crimea, and Countries Adjacent to the Black Sea in the Years 1835–36* (London, 1855)

Ross, J., *Three Generations of Englishwomen. Memoirs and Correspondence of Mrs. John Taylor, Mrs. Sarah Austin, and Lady Duff Gordon*, 2 vols (London, 1888)

Rousseau, J.-J., *Les Confessions*, new ed. (Paris, n.d.)

Russell, J., *Journal of a Tour in Ceylon and India, Undertaken at the Request of the Baptist Missionary Society, in Company with the Rev. J. Leechman, M.A., with Observations and Remarks* (London, 1852)

Russell, P., *A Treatise on the Plague . . .* (London, 1791)

Sainte-Maure, C. de, *A New Journey through Greece, Ægypt, Palestine, Italy, Swisserland, Alsatia, and the Netherlands . . .* (London, 1725)

Salle, E. de, *Pérégrinations en Orient ou Voyage pittoresque, historique et politique en Egypte, Nubie, Syrie, Turquie, Grèce pendant les Années 1837–38–39*, 2 vols (Paris, 1840)

Sanderson, J., *The Travels of John Sanderson in the Levant 1584–1602 . . . Edited by Sir William Foster . . .*, Series II, 67 vols (Hakluyt Society, London, 1931)

Sandwich, *A Voyage Performed by the Late Earl of Sandwich Round the Mediterranean in the Years 1738 and 1739. Written by Himself . . .* (London, 1799)

Sandys, G., *Sandys Travels, Containing an History of the Original and Present State of the Turkish Empire . . .*, 7th ed. (London, 1673)

Saulcy, F. de, *Narrative of a Journey Round the Dead Sea and in the Bible Lands in 1850 and 1851*, 2 vols (London, 1853)

Saumery, P.L. de, *Memoires et Avantures Secretes et Curieuses d'un Voyage du Levant par Mr. De Mirone [pseudonym]*, 6 vols in three (Liège, 1732–5)

Schwartz, M.E. von, *Leaves from a Lady's Diary of her Travels in Barbary*, 2 vols (London, 1850)

Scott, C. Rochfort, *Rambles in Egypt and Candia . . .*, 2 vols (London, 1837)

Scott, C.H., *The Baltic, the Black Sea, and the Crimea . . .*, 2nd ed. (London, 1854)

Scott, W., *Life of Sir Walter Scott, Bart: Begun by Himself . . .*, Lockhart, J.G. (ed.), 3rd ed. (Edinburgh, 1853)

Scott, W., *Memoirs of Sir Walter Scott*, 5 vols (Macmillan, London, 1900)

Semple, R., *Observations on a Journey Through Spain and Italy to Naples; and Thence to Smyrna and Constantinople . . .*, 2nd ed., 2 vols (London, 1808)

Senior, N.W., *Journals Kept in France and Italy from 1848 to 1852 . . . Edited by His Daughter M.C.M. Simpson*, 2 vols (London, 1871)

Sherer, J.M., *Scenes and Impressions in Egypt and in Italy*, 2nd ed. (London, 1825)

Sheil, Lady M.L., *Glimpses of Life and Manners in Persia* (London, 1856)

Simpson, J.P., *Letters from the Danube*, 2 vols (London, 1847)

Sinclair, J.D., *An Autumn in Italy, Being a Personal Narrative of a Tour in the Austrian, Tuscan, Roman and Sardinian States, in 1827* (Edinburgh and London, 1829)

Skene, J.H., *The Frontier Lands of the Christian and the Turk; Comprising Travels in the Regions of the Lower Danube, in 1850 and 1851 . . .*, 2nd ed., 2 vols (London, 1853)

Slade, A., *Turkey, Greece and Malta*, 2 vols (London, 1837)

Slade, A., *Travels in Germany and Russia: Including a Steam Voyage by the Danube and the Euxine from Vienna to Constantinople, in 1838–39* (London, 1840)

Slade, A., *Records of Travels in Turkey, Greece, etc. and of a Cruise in the Black Sea with the Capitan Pacha*, new ed. (London, 1854)

Smith, A., *A Month at Constantinople*, 2nd ed. (London, 1850)

Snow, R., *Journal of a Steam Voyage Down the Danube to Constantinople, and Thence by Way of Malta and Marseilles to England* (London, 1842)

Spencer, E., *Travels in Circassia, Krim Tartary, &c. Including a Steam Voyage Down the Danube, from Vienna to Constantinople and Round the Black Sea, in 1836*, 2 vols (London, 1837)

Spencer, E., *Travels in the Western Caucasus, Including a Tour Through Imeritia, Mingrelia, Turkey, Moldavia, Galicia, Silesia, and Moravia, in 1836*, 2 vols (London, 1838)

Spencer, E., *Travels in European Turkey, in 1850, Through Bosnia, Servia, Bulgaria, Macedonia, Thrace, Albania, and Epirus; with a Visit to Greece and the Ionian Isles . . .*, 2 vols (London, 1851)

Spencer, J.A., *Sketches of Travels in Egypt and the Holy Land* (London, 1850)

Spon, J. & Whe[e]ler, G., *Voyage D'Italie, de Dalmatie, de Grece, et du Levant, fait és années 1675 & 1676*, 2 vols (Amsterdam, 1679)

Spry, W.J.J., *Life on the Bosphorus . . .* (London, 1895)

Stanford's Compendium of Geography & Travel (London, 1885)

Starke, M., *Information and Directions for Travellers on the Continent*, 6th ed. (London, 1828)

Starke, M., *Travels on the Continent: Written for the Use and Particular Information of Travellers* (London, 1820)

Starke, M., *Travels in Europe, for the Use of Travellers on the Continent . . .*, 9th ed. (Paris, 1839)

Stendhal Beyle, M.H., *pseudonym* Stendhal, *Memoirs D'Un Touriste . . .*, 3 vols (Gallimard, Paris, 1932)

Stent, W. Drew, *Egypt and the Holy Land in 1842, with Sketches of Greece, Constantinople, and the Levant*, 2 vols (London, 1843)

Stephens, J.L., *Incidents of Travel in the Russian and Turkish Empires*, 2 vols (London, 1839)

Strickland, H.E., *Memoirs of Hugh Edwin Strickland, M.A . . .*, Jardine, Sir W. (ed.) (London, 1858)

Stuart, Lt. Colonel [C.], *Journal of a Residence in Northern Persia and the Adjacent Provinces of Turkey* (London, 1854)

Sutherland, Capt. D., *A Tour Up the Straits, from Gibraltar to Constantinople . . .*, 2nd ed. (London, 1790)

Swan, Revd C., *Journal of a Voyage Up the Mediterranean; Principally Among the Islands of the Archipelago, and in Asia Minor. . .*, 2 vols (London, 1826)

Tafur, P., *Travels and Adventures 1435–1439 Translated and Edited with an Introduction by Malcolm Letts* (London, 1926)
Taylor, B., *Pictures of Palestine, Asia Minor, Sicily, and Spain; or, the Lands of the Saracen* (London, 1855)
Tchihatchef, P. de, *Le Bosphore et Constantinople* . . ., 2nd ed. (Paris, 1866)
Temple, Major Sir G., *Travels in Greece and Turkey Being the Second Part of Excursions in the Mediterranean*, 2 vols in one (London, 1836)
Temple, Revd D. H., *Life and Letters of Rev. Daniel Temple, for Twenty-Three Years a Missionary for the A.B.C.F.M. in Western Asia* . . . (Boston, 1855)
Teonge, H., *The Diary of Henry Teonge Chaplain on Board H.M.'s Ships Assistance, Bristol, and Royal Oak 1675–1679*, Manwaring, G.E. (ed.) (London, 1927)
Terry, C., *Scenes and Thoughts in Foreign Lands* (London, 1848)
Tets, H.R. van, *Voyage d'une Hollandaise en France en 1819* (Paris, 1966)
Thackeray, W.M., *Notes of a Journey from Cornhill to Grand Cairo, by Way of Lisbon, Athens, Constantinople, and Jerusalem* . . ., Titmarsh, M.A. (pseudonym) (London, 1846)
Thévenot, *Relation d'un Voyage fait au Levant . . . Par Monsieur Thévenot* (Paris, 1664)
Thielmann, M. von, *Journey in The Caucasus, Persia and Turkey in Asia*, Heneage, Charles (trans.), 2 vols (London, 1875)
Thomson, W.M., *The Land and the Book* . . ., 2 vols (New York, 1859)
Ticknor Hillard, G.S. (ed.), *Life, Letters, and Journals of George Ticknor*, 2 vols (Boston, 1876)
Tischendorff, C., *Travels in the East . . . translated from the German by W.E. Shuckard* (London, 1847)
Tobin, C., *Shadows of the East; or Slight Sketches of Scenery, Persons, and Customs, from Observations During a Tour in 1853 and 1854, in Egypt, Palestine, Syria, Turkey, and Greece* (London, 1855)
Tournefort, J. Pitton de, *A Voyage into the Levant: Perform'd by Command of the Late French King* . . ., 2 vols (London, 1718)
Trant Luard, C.G. (ed.), *The Journal of Clarissa Trant 1800–1832* (Bodley Head, London, 1925)
Trant, Capt. T. Abercromby, *Narrative of a Journey Through Greece, in 1830* . . . (London, 1830)
Tully, R., *Letters Written During a Ten Years' Residence at the Court of Tripoli* . . . (London, 1819)
Turner, W., *Journal of a Tour in the Levant*, 3 vols (London, 1820)
Twain, M., *The Innocents Abroad, or the New Pilgrims' Progress* . . ., Clemens, Samuel L. (ed.) (Hartford, 1875)
Twain, M., *Travelling with the Innocents Abroad: Mark Twain's Original Reports from Europe and the Holy Land*, McKeithan, D.M. (ed.) (University of Oklahoma, Norman, 1958)
Urquhart, D., *The Pillars of Hercules; or, a Narrative of Travels in Spain and Morocco in 1848*, 2 vols (London, 1850)
Usborne, T.H., *New Guide to the Levant* . . . (London, 1840)
Valery, M., *Historical, Literary, and Artistical Travels in Italy*, Clifton, C.E. (trans.) (Paris, 1839)
Valle, P. della, *Les Fameux Voyages de Pietro Della Valle, Gentil-homme Romain, surnommé L'Illustre Voyageur* . . ., 4 vols (Paris, 1664)

Valle, P. della, *Voyages de Pietro Della Valle, Gentilhomme Romain . . . nouvelle édition . . .*, 8 vols (Rouen, 1745)

Vane, F.A. [Londonderry, Marchioness of], *Narrative of a Visit to the Courts of Vienna, Constantinople, Athens, Naples, &c.* (London, 1844)

Vane, C.W. [Londonderry, Marquess of], *A Steam Voyage to Constantinople, by the Rhine and the Danube, in 1840–41, and to Portugal, Spain, &c., in 1839 . . .*, 2 vols (London, 1842)

Veryard, E., *An Account of Divers Choice Remarks, . . . Taken in a Journey Through the Low-Countries, France, Italy and Part of Spain; with the Isles of Sicily and Malta as also, a Voyage to the Levant . . .* (London, 1701)

Vigier, Le Vicomte R., *Un Parisien à Constantinople* (Paris, 1886)

Walpole, Lt. the Hon. F., R.N., *The Ansayrii, and the Assassins, with Travels in the Further East in 1850–51, Including a Visit to Nineveh*, 3 vols (London, 1851)

Walsh, Revd R., *Narrative of a Journey from Constantinople to England*, 3rd ed. (London, 1829)

Warburton, E., *The Crescent and the Cross; or, Romance and Realities of Eastern Travel . . .*, 2 vols (London, 1845)

Waring, G., *Letters from Malta and Sicily Addressed to a Young Naturalist* (London, 1843)

Watson, W., *A Cruise in the Aegean . . .* (London, 1853)

Wilbraham, Capt. R., *Travels in the Trans-Caucasian Provinces of Russia, and Along the Southern Shore of the Lakes of Van and Urumiah, in the Autumn and Winter of 1837* (London, 1839)

Wilde, W.R., *Narrative of a Voyage to Madeira, Teneriffe, and Along the Shores of the Mediterranean . . .*, 2 vols (Dublin and London, 1840)

Wilkinson, C., *A Tour Through Asia Minor and the Greek Islands . . .* (London, 1806)

Wilkinson, Sir G., *Hand-Book for Travellers in Egypt . . .* (London, 1847)

Wilkinson, Sir G., *Modern Egypt and Thebes . . .*, 2 vols (London, 1843)

Willis, N.P., *Pencillings by the Way*, new ed. (London, 1850)

Wilson, J., *The Lands of the Bible Visited and Described . . .*, 2 vols (Edinburgh, London and Dublin, 1847)

Wilson, Revd S.S., *A Narrative of the Greek Mission; or Sixteen Years in Malta and Greece . . .* (London, 1839)

Wilson, W.R., *Travels in Egypt and the Holy Land . . . with a Journey Through Turkey, Greece, the Ionian Islands, Sicily, Spain, &c.* (London, 1824)

Wittman, W., *Travels in Turkey, Asia-Minor, Syria, and Across the Desert into Egypt During the Years 1799, 1800, and 1801 . . .* (London, 1803)

Wolff, Revd Dr J., *Narrative of a Mission to Bokhara, in the Years 1843–1845, to Ascertain the Fate of Colonel Stoddart and Captain Conolly*, 5th ed. (Edinburgh and London, 1848)

Woodruff, S., *Journal of a Tour to Malta, Greece, Asia Minor, Carthage, Algiers, Port Mahon, and Spain, in 1828 . . .* (Hartford, 1831)

Woods, J., *Letters of an Architect, from France, Italy, and Greece*, 2 vols (London, 1828)

Young, C.G., *A Wayfarer's Notes on the Shores of the Levant, and the Valley of the Nile. . .* (Edinburgh, 1848)

Secondary sources

Barnes, D.S., 'Cargo, "Infection", and the Logic of Quarantine in the Nineteenth Century' in *Bulletin of the History of Medicine*, vol. 88, no. 1 (Spring 2014), 75–100

Bates, E.S., *Touring in 1600* (London, 1911; republished by Century, London, 1987)

Black, J., *The British Abroad: The Grand Tour in the Eighteenth Century* (Alan Sutton, Stroud; St. Martin's Press, New York, 1992)

Booker, J., *Maritime Quarantine: The British Experience, c. 1650–1900* (Ashgate, Aldershot, 2007, now Routledge)

Brennan, N.G. (ed.), *The Origins of the Grand Tour . . .*, Series III, 14 vols (Hakluyt Society, London, 2004)

Carrington, D., *The Traveller's Eye* (The Pilot Press, London, 1947)

Cassar, P., *Medical History of Malta* (Wellcome Historical Medical Library, London, 1965)

Chessell, C.I., 'Britain's Ionian Consul: Spiridion Foresti and the Return to the Islands 1807–1810' in *Journal of Mediterranean Studies*, vol. 19, no. 2 (January 2010), 201–18

Cox, E.G., *A Reference Guide to the Literature of Travel . . .*, 3 vols (University of Washington, Seattle, 1948–50)

Fedden, R., *English Travellers in the Near East* (Longmans, Green & Co., for The British Council, London, New York and Toronto, 1958)

Gibson, E.C.S., *John Howard* (Harper Bros, London, 1901)

Harrison, M., *Contagion: How Commerce Has Spread Disease* (Yale University Press, New Haven and London, 2013)

Healy, M., 'Highways, Hospitals and Boundary Hazards' in Betteridge, T. (ed.), *Borders and Travellers in Early Modern Europe* (Ashgate, Aldershot, 2007)

Henderson, J., *The Renaissance Hospital: Healing the Body and Healing the Soul* (Yale University Press, New Haven and London, 2006)

Herlihy, P., *Odessa: A History* (Harvard University Press, Cambridge, MA, 1986)

Hibbert, C., *The Grand Tour* (Thames Methuen, London, 1987)

Huxley, G., *Lady Elizabeth and the Grosvenors: Life in a Whig Family, 1822–1839* (Oxford University Press, London, New York and Toronto, 1965)

Macaulay, D., 'The Little Red Flag, Part 2, Syra' in *Pratique, Newsletter*, vol. 2 (1976), 17–18

Norwich, J.J., *A Taste for Travel* (Macmillan, London, 1985)

Panzac, D., *Quarantaines et Lazarets. L'Europe et la Peste d'Orient (XVIIe – XXe Siècles)* (Aix en Provence, Edisud, 1986)

Paris, R., *Histoire du Commerce de Marseille . . .*, 5 vols (Librairie Plon, Paris, 1949–57)

Risse, G.B., *Mending Bodies, Saving Souls: A History of Hospitals* (Oxford University Press, New York and Oxford, 1999)

Slatter, E.M., 'The New Lazaretto at Siros (Syra), Greece, in 1840' in *Medical History*, vol. 28 (1984), 73–80

Starkey, P. & Starkey, J. (eds.), *Travellers in Egypt* (I.B.Tauris, London and New York, 1998)

Sultana, D., *Benjamin Disraeli in Spain, Malta and Albania 1830–32. A Monograph* (Tamesis Books, London, 1976)

Sultana, D., *The Journey of Sir Walter Scott to Malta* (St. Martin's Press, Gloucester and New York, 1986)
Trease, G., *The Grand Tour* (Heineman, London, 1967)
Trethewey, R., *Mistress of the Arts* (Headline, London, 2002)
Vandervelde, V.D., 'Russia: The Disinfection of Mail: Early Documentary Sources' in *Pratique, Newsletter*, vol. 2 (Winter 1974–5), 22–7
Weber, S.H., *Voyages and Travels in the Near East Made During the XIX Century. . .* (American School of Classical Studies at Athens, Princeton, NJ, 1952)
Weber, S.H., *Voyages and Travels in Greece, the Near East and Adjacent Regions Made Previous to the Year 1801. . .* (American School of Classical Studies at Athens, Princeton, NJ, 1953)

Index

www.ingramcontent.com/pod-product-compliance
Lightning Source LLC
LaVergne TN
LVHW021126300926
849160LV00010B/875

* 9 7 8 1 0 3 2 0 5 0 3 5 5 *